RENAL AND UROLOGIC DISORDERS

URETROSCOPIC LITHOTRIPSY

THE IDEAL TREATMENT OF UROLITHIASIS

RENAL AND UROLOGIC DISORDERS

Additional books in this series can be found on Nova's website under the Series tab.

Additional e-books in this series can be found on Nova's website under the e-book tab.

RENAL AND UROLOGIC DISORDERS

URETROSCOPIC LITHOTRIPSY

THE IDEAL TREATMENT OF UROLITHIASIS

RYOJI TAKAZAWA, M.D., PH.D.
TAKASHI KAWAHARA, M.D.
JUNICHI MATSUZAKI, M.D., PH.D.
HIROKI ITO, M.D.
TETSUO YOSHIKAWA, M.D., PH.D.
SACHI KITAYAMA, M.D.
AND
TOSHIHIKO TSUJII, M.D., PH.D.

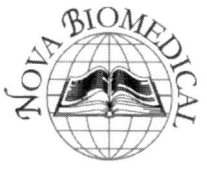

New York

Copyright © 2014 by Nova Science Publishers, Inc.

All rights reserved. No part of this book may be reproduced, stored in a retrieval system or transmitted in any form or by any means: electronic, electrostatic, magnetic, tape, mechanical photocopying, recording or otherwise without the written permission of the Publisher.

For permission to use material from this book please contact us:
Telephone 631-231-7269; Fax 631-231-8175
Web Site: http://www.novapublishers.com

NOTICE TO THE READER

The Publisher has taken reasonable care in the preparation of this book, but makes no expressed or implied warranty of any kind and assumes no responsibility for any errors or omissions. No liability is assumed for incidental or consequential damages in connection with or arising out of information contained in this book. The Publisher shall not be liable for any special, consequential, or exemplary damages resulting, in whole or in part, from the readers' use of, or reliance upon, this material. Any parts of this book based on government reports are so indicated and copyright is claimed for those parts to the extent applicable to compilations of such works.

Independent verification should be sought for any data, advice or recommendations contained in this book. In addition, no responsibility is assumed by the publisher for any injury and/or damage to persons or property arising from any methods, products, instructions, ideas or otherwise contained in this publication.

This publication is designed to provide accurate and authoritative information with regard to the subject matter covered herein. It is sold with the clear understanding that the Publisher is not engaged in rendering legal or any other professional services. If legal or any other expert assistance is required, the services of a competent person should be sought. FROM A DECLARATION OF PARTICIPANTS JOINTLY ADOPTED BY A COMMITTEE OF THE AMERICAN BAR ASSOCIATION AND A COMMITTEE OF PUBLISHERS.

Additional color graphics may be available in the e-book version of this book.

Library of Congress Cataloging-in-Publication Data

ISBN: 978-1-63117-922-8

Library of Congress Control Number: 2014941042

Published by Nova Science Publishers, Inc. † New York

Contents

Preface		vii
PART I. INDICATIONS		1
Chapter 1	Indications for Ureteroscopic Lithotripsy *Ryoji Takazawa, M.D., Ph.D.,* *Sachi Kitayama, M.D.* *and Toshihiko Tsujii, M.D., Ph.D.*	3
PART II. INSTRUMENTATION		17
Chapter 2	Instrumentation for Ureteroscopic Lithotripsy *Ryoji Takazawa, M.D., Ph.D.,* *Sachi Kitayama, M.D.* *and Toshihiko Tsujii, M.D., Ph.D.*	19
PART III. TECHNIQUES		51
Chapter 3	Preoperative Preparation: Antibiotics, Prestenting, and Percutaneous Nephrostomy *Takashi Kawahara, M.D., Hiroki Ito, M.D.,* *Hiroji Uemura, M.D., Ph.D.,* *Yoshinobu Kubota, M.D., Ph.D.,* *Junichi Matsuzaki, M.D., Ph.D.*	53
Chapter 4	Semirigid and Flexible Ureteroscopy: Ohtsuka Method *Ryoji Takazawa, M.D., Ph.D.,* *Sachi Kitayama, M.D.* *and Toshihiko Tsujii, M.D., Ph.D.*	63

vi Contents

Chapter 5	Semirigid and Flexible Ureteroscopy: Ohguchi-Higashi Method *Junichi Matsuzaki, M.D., Ph.D.,* *Takashi Kawahara, M.D.,* *Hiroki Ito, M.D.,* *Hiroji Uemura, M.D., Ph.D.,* *Masahiro Yao, M.D., Ph.D.* *and Yoshinobu Kubota, M.D., Ph.D.*	77
Chapter 6	Stenting and Postoperative Care *Takashi Kawahara, M.D.,* *Hiroki Ito, M.D.,* *Hiroji Uemura, M.D., Ph.D.,* *Yoshinobu Kubota, M.D., Ph.D.* *and Junichi Matsuzaki, M.D., Ph.D.*	87
Chapter 7	Combination with PCNL: Ureteroscopy-Assisted Retrograde Nephrostomy (UARN) *Takashi Kawahara, M.D., Hiroki Ito, M.D.,* *Hiroji Uemura, M.D., Ph.D.,* *Yoshinobu Kubota, M.D., Ph.D.* *and Junichi Matsuzaki, M.D., Ph.D.*	99
PART IV. EVALUATIONS		**111**
Chapter 8	Pre- and Post-Operative Evaluations *Hiroki Ito, M.D., Takashi Kawahara, M.D.,* *Masahiro Yao, M.D., Ph.D., Yoshinobu Kubota,* *M.D., Ph.D. and Junichi Matsuzaki, M.D., Ph.D.*	113
Chapter 9	Complications of Ureteroscopy *Tetsuo Yoshikawa, M.D., Ph.D.*	127
Chapter 10	Evidence for Staged Operations *Ryoji Takazawa, M.D., Ph.D.,* *Sachi Kitayama, M.D.* *and Toshihiko Tsujii, M.D., Ph.D.*	133
POSTFACE: FUTURE VISION		**141**
Authors' Contact Information		**145**
Index		**147**

Preface

The clinical management of urolithiasis is now in a new era of ureteroscopic lithotripsy. Ureteroscopic lithotripsy has become an effective and safe treatment for both renal and ureteral stones, and its indications have been expanding. The advantages of ureteroscopy over shock-wave lithotripsy are its ability to directly access stones throughout the entire urinary collecting system either unilaterally or bilaterally, and to actively remove stone fragments. For large renal stones, percutaneous nephrolithotomy is now a standard treatment, but its major complication rates are not negligible. Ureteroscopic lithotripsy is a type of endoscopic surgery that is performed through the natural orifice, which thus avoids the onset of any renal parenchymal damage. New surgical techniques which combine percutaneous and transurethral approaches have been developed. Ureteroscopes and their working devices have rapidly improved, and further improvements will lead to even better outcomes in the next decade.

Ureteroscopic Lithotripsy: The ideal Treatment of Urolithiasis presents the latest knowledge and the skills used for ureteroscopic surgery for urolithiasis. It consists of four sections (Indications, Instrumentations, Techniques and Evaluations). This book provides essential information for urologists who want to learn the techniques of this type of endourological surgery.

Ryoji Takazawa, M.D., Ph.D.

PART I. INDICATIONS

Chapter 1

Indications for Ureteroscopic Lithotripsy

Ryoji Takazawa*, *M.D., Ph.D., Sachi Kitayama, M.D.
and Toshihiko Tsujii, M.D., Ph.D.*
Department of Urology, Tokyo Metropolitan Ohtsuka Hospital,
Tokyo, Japan

Abstract

The technical developments in and patient requests for rapid stone removal have led to changes in clinical stone management. The demand for imperative complete stone removal has led to a shift toward endourology. For kidney stones, we recommend endoscopic treatment, because residual fragments after shock wave lithotripsy (SWL) are not easy to pass spontaneously, and often lead to recurrent stone formation. Kidney stones measuring up to 40 mm in size can be treated by flexible ureteroscopy (URS) monotherapy, although staged procedures may be required. We also recommend using a combination of percutaneous nephrolithotomy (PCNL) and flexible URS for larger stones, especially for staghorn stones, because URS can access each calyx where the percutaneous antegrade approach is difficult. For ureteral stones, URS or

---

[*] Corresponding author: Ryoji Takazawa, M.D., Ph.D. ryoji_takazawa@tmhp.jp.

SWL are common first-line recommended treatment options with no distinction with regard to the stone position.

Introduction

The technical developments in and patient requests for rapid stone removal have led to changes in clinical stone management. In the past 30 years, stone treatment has shifted from open surgery to percutaneous surgery, and this was almost replaced by shock wave lithotripsy (SWL). However, during the last decade, the limitations of SWL for some situations became evident, and ureteroscopy (URS) has become more available. The demand for imperative complete stone removal has led to a shift toward endourology. The ureteroscopes and related instruments are still evolving. This evolution has enabled the treatment of urinary stones in all locations, while decreasing the morbidity associated with the active intervention.

1. Indications for Active Treatment

In general, there is a consensus that small stones may be treated with conservative management. For ureteral stones of 10 mm or less, spontaneous passage is seen in many patients. Spontaneous passages are observed in 68% of patients with < 5 mm stones, and in 47% of patients with > 5 mm stones [1]. For patients with < 10 mm ureteral stones, a period of observation is appropriate in the absence of complicating factors such as infection, renal dysfunction or poor pain control. However, observation for longer than four to six weeks is generally not advised due to the negative effects on renal function, although the precise duration of observation has not been well defined [2]. In a patient who has a newly diagnosed ureteral stone < 10 mm and if active stone removal is not indicated, observation with periodic evaluation is considered to be an option for initial treatment.

Most kidney stones are asymptomatic, and it is questionable for small stones, especially in the lower pole, if treatment is required. The natural history and the risk of progression of such calculi have not been well evaluated. However, stone growth, potential obstruction, associated infection and pain are clear indications for the treatment of such stones. Several authors have reported a significant rate of incidents during the follow-up of renal calyceal stones (Table 1).

Table 1. The natural history of asymptomatic caliceal stones

Authors (year)	Study type	No. of patients	Follow-up	Disease progression (stone growth)	Symptomatic episode	Need for intervention
Glowacki et al. (1992)	Retrospective	107	31.6 months	n. a.	31.8%	16.8%
Hubner et al. (1990)	Retrospective	80	7.4 years	45%	68%	83%
Keeley et al. (2001)	Randomized prospective	200	2.2 years	n. a.	21%	10%
Burgher et al. (2004)	Retrospective	300	3.26 years	77%	n. a.	26%
Inci et al. (2007)	Retrospective	24	52.3 months	33.3%	41.7%	11%

For example, Glowacki et al. have reported that symptomatic events developed in 31.8% of patients, and spontaneous passage occurred in 15.0%, while surgical interventions were required in 16.8% [3]. In a recent retrospective study, Burgher et al. reported that 77% of asymptomatic patients with renal stones experienced disease progression, with 26% requiring surgical intervention [4]. In a retrospective study, Hubner and Porpaczy reported that an infection developed in 68% of patients with asymptomatic calyceal stones, and 45% had an increase in stone size after 7.4 years of follow-up. They also suggested that 83% of calyceal calculi require intervention within the first five years after the diagnosis [5]. Finally, Inci et al. have investigated lower pole calyceal stones, and observed that within a follow-up period of 52.3 months, nine (33.3%) patients had increased stone size, while only three (11%) patients required intervention [6]. In a prospective randomized controlled trial with a 2.2-year clinical follow-up, Keeley et al. have reported no significant difference between SWL and observation when they compared patients with asymptomatic calyceal stones < 15 mm in terms of the stone-free rate, symptoms, requirement for additional treatment, quality of life, renal function and the hospital admission rate [7]. Although some authors have recommended prophylactic treatment for these asymptomatic kidney stones, conflicting data have been reported in the literature on this subject [8].

In contrast to renal stones, ureteral stones usually cause symptoms, such as acute renal colic. Intervention is required when symptoms are not manageable and spontaneous passage is unlikely, even with medical expulsive therapy (MET). Persistent pain, renal insufficiency or a solitary kidney and emerging urosepsis are other situations where timely intervention is mandatory. Other indications for active stone removal are shown in Table 2.

Table 2. The indications for active stone removal

Ureteral stones	Kidney stones
Low likelihood of spontaneous passage (stone size >7-8 mm, proximal stone location)	Stone growth
Persistent pain despite adequate analgesic medication	Patients at high risk for stone formation
Persistent obstruction	Obstruction caused by stones
Renal insufficiency (e.g. renal failure, bilateral obstruction, single kidney)	Infection
Infection	Symptomatic stones (e.g. pain, macrohematuria)
	Stones ≥15 mm
	Stones <15 mm if observation is not the option of choice
	Patient preference
	Comorbidity
	Social situation of the patient (e.g. profession or travelling)

2. Selection of the Procedure for Active Removal of Kidney Stones

2.1. Stones in the Renal Pelvis or Upper/Middle Calices

The minimally invasive treatment options for renal calculi include SWL, percutaneous nephrolithotomy (PCNL) or flexible URS. Laparoscopic and open approaches are limited to selected situations, i.e., in cases with concomitant problems, such as ureteropelvic junction (UPJ) obstruction, that have to be corrected simultaneously. While the efficacy of PCNL is not affected by the stone size, the stone-free rates (SFRs) of SWL and URS decrease with stone size.

SWL achieves a good SFR for stones up to 20 mm at all intrarenal locations, except for the lower pole and diverticula. Therefore, SWL remains the method of choice for such stones according to most guidelines [9].

In the last decade, endoscopic procedures (PCNL, flexible URS) have also achieved excellent SFRs. Stones > 20 mm should be treated by PCNL primarily. If necessary, PCNL should be combined with flexible URS. A synchronous approach with PCNL and URS with the patient in the Galdakao-modified Valdivia position or prone split-leg position has been suggested to be useful [10, 11].

Flexible URS has been demonstrated to be effective for renal stones. For larger stones (> 20 mm), URS monotherapy has also achieved an excellent SFR, although its outcome depends on the operator's skills and it may require staged procedures [12-15]. In our recent experience, flexible URS has been a favorable option for larger renal stones (20-40 mm) [15]. We reported a 100% SFR for stones 20-40 mm by an average of 1.3 procedures, compared with a SFR for stones > 40 mm of 67% after an average of 1.8 procedures. Although PCNL is currently the first-line recommended treatment for patients with renal stones > 20 mm, its major complication rate is not negligible, and less invasive approaches, including flexible URS, need to be explored.

2.2. Stones in the Lower Renal Pole

Although the disintegration efficacy of SWL is not limited compared to that in other locations, the SFR for stones in the lower renal pole is worse than that in other intrarenal locations, because the fragments often remain in the calyx and lead to recurrent stone formation. The reported SFR of SWL for lower pole calculi is 25-85% [16-21]. Apart from the stone size and composition, other factors, including a steep infundibular-pelvic angle, long calyx (> 10 mm) and a narrow infundibulum (<5 mm), negatively influence the SFR after SWL [22-28].

Therefore, endourological procedures are preferred as the primary treatment for stones in the lower renal pole. PCNL is recommended for stones > 20 mm in the lower renal pole. PCNL might be a reasonable alternative even for smaller calculi if other treatment options are not feasible. Based on the available comparative literature, flexible URS seems to have comparable efficacy to SWL [20, 21]. However, several recently published case series and our own experience suggested that flexible URS has a clear advantage over SWL [12-15].

2.3. Our Current Proposal for Active Removal of Kidney Stones

Figure 1 shows our proposed treatment algorithm for kidney stones, in comparison to the 2013 EAU guidelines. We select the treatment option with no distinction regarding the stone position (upper/middle pole or lower pole); because the current URS instruments can easily approach all calyces, including the lower calyx, and can actively remove the stone fragments by using a basket. Basically, we recommend endoscopic treatment for kidney stones, because residual fragments after SWL frequently do not pass spontaneously and often lead to recurrent stone formation. Depending on the operator's skills and the stone shape/position, stones up to 40 mm can be treated sufficiently by flexible URS monotherapy, although staged procedures may be required. We also recommend the combination of PCNL and flexible URS for larger stones, especially for staghorn stones, because the URS can access each calyx where the percutaneous antegrade approach is difficult. This is associated with a major advantage in terms of clearing the stone burden [10, 11]. Multi-tract PCNL has also been evaluated by experts, who reported successful outcomes. However, multi-tract procedures may cause more complications, but if necessary, should be considered for appropriate cases [28, 29].

Ureteral calculi are usually treated by SWL or retrograde URS. Laparoscopic or open surgery is invasive and should be reserved for special cases. Another alternative approach for selected cases is percutaneous antegrade removal of ureteral stones. Antegrade URS might therefore be a good option for large impacted stones in the proximal ureter or when retrograde access is not possible, e.g., after urinary diversion.

3.1. Proximal Ureteral Stones

Based on a large meta-analysis performed by the American Urological Association (AUA) and the European Association of Urology (EAU), no difference in the overall SFR could be detected between SWL and URS for proximal stones [1]. However, after stratifying patients for stone size, SWL had a higher SFR for stones < 10 mm than URS, while URS was superior for stones > 10 mm (Table 3). This difference could be explained by the SFR for URS, which did not vary significantly with size, whereas the SFR following SWL was negatively correlated with the stone size.

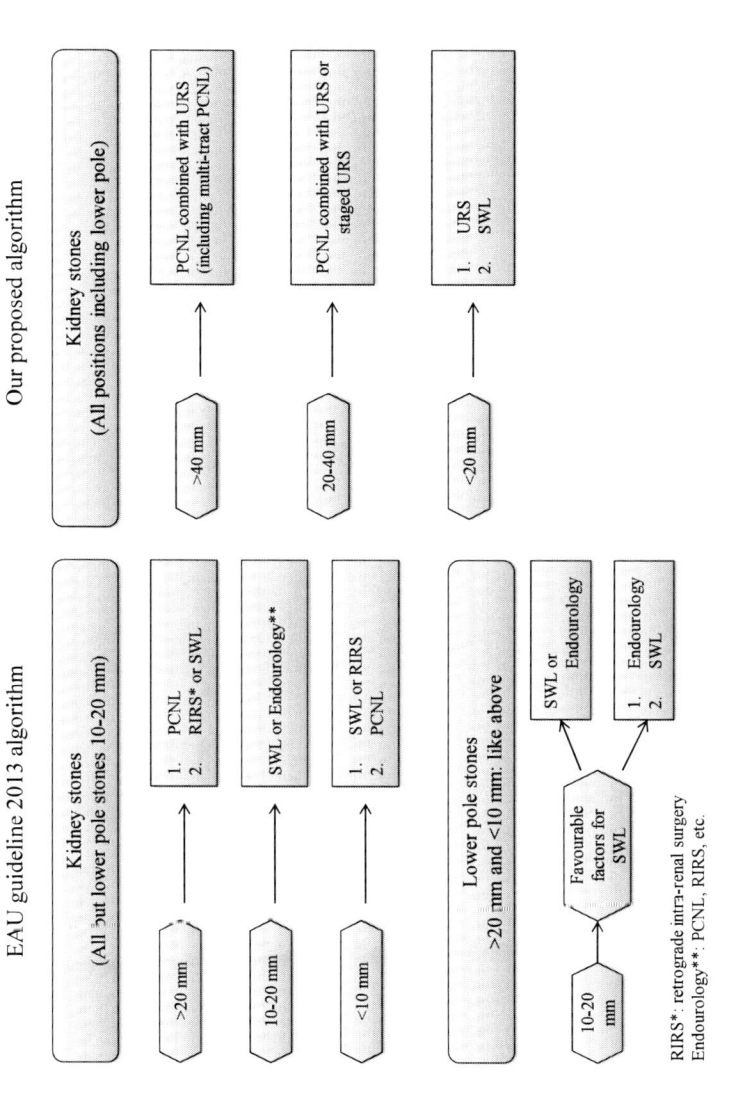

Figure 1. The treatment algorithm for kidney stones.

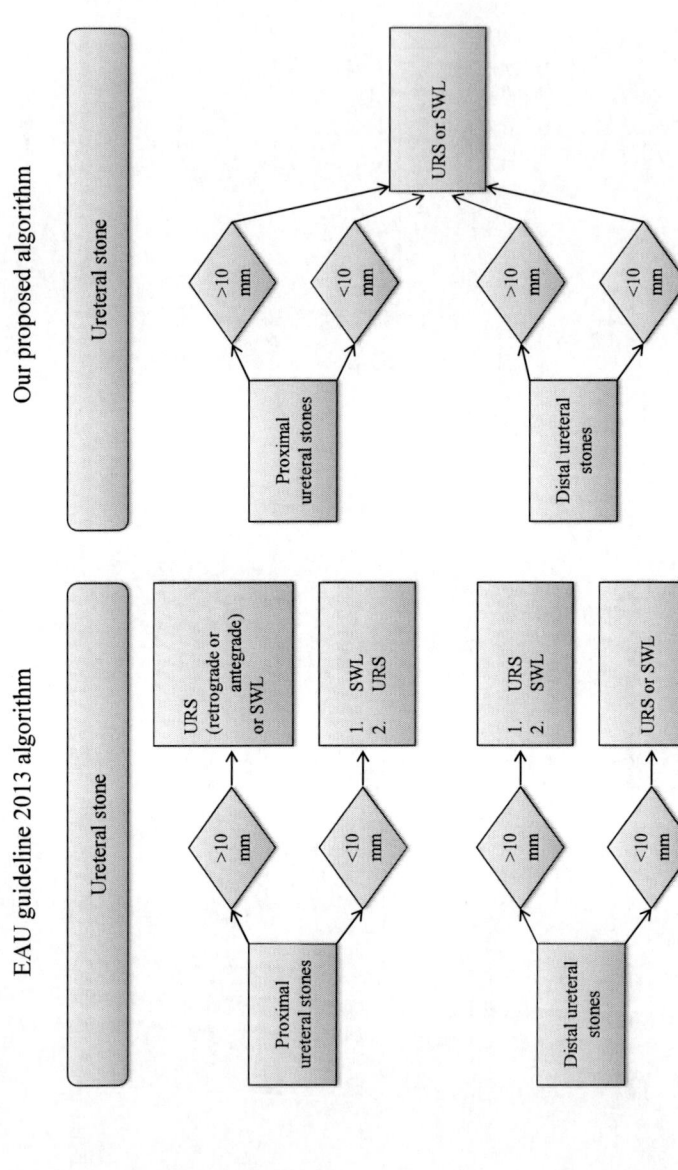

Figure 2. The treatment algorithm for ureteral stones.

According to the EAU-AUA meta-analysis, patients should be informed that URS is associated with a better chance of achieving stone-free status with a single procedure, but that is also associated with a higher complication rate. However, the European practice of using semirigid URS for proximal stones has proven to be safe and effective [30].

Although there is insufficient data available to statistically compare flexible and semirigid URS for proximal ureteral stones, favorable SFRs have been reported using flexible URS (87%) compared with rigid or semirigid (77%) URS [1]. The SFRs will probably continue to improve as the distribution and further technical improvement of flexible URS continues.

3. Selection of the Procedure for the Active Removal of Ureteral Stones

3.2. Mid- and Distal Ureteral Stones

For all mid-ureteral stones, URS appears to be superior to SWL, but after stratification for stone size, the small number of patients limited the statistical significance. For all distal stones, URS yielded a better overall SFR compared to SWL, independent of the stone size (Table 3).

Table 3. The stone-free rates after primary SWL or URS treatment for ureteral stones

Stone location and size	SWL		URS	
	No. of patients	SFR% (95% CI)	No. of patients	SFR% (95% CI)
Distal ureter	7217	74% (73-75)	10372	93% (93-94)
<10 mm	1684	86% (80-91)	2013	97% (96-98)
>10 mm	966	74% (57-87)	668	93% (91-95)
Mid ureter	1697	73% (71-75)	1140	87% (85-89)
<10 mm	44	84% (65-95)	116	93% (88-98)
>10 mm	15	76% (36-97)	110	79% (71-87)
Proximal ureter	6682	82% (81-83)	2448	82% (81-84)
<10 mm	967	89% (87-91)	318	84% (80-88)
>10 mm	481	70% (66-74)	338	81% (77-85)

3.3. Our Current Proposal for the Active Removal of Ureteral Stones

Figure 2 shows our proposed treatment algorithm for ureteral stones, in comparison with the 2013 EAU guidelines. Ureteroscopic lithotripsy has become a first-line recommended treatment for all ureteral stones in any location. Thus, URS and SWL are the most common treatment options for ureteral stones, with no distinction regarding the stone position.

4. Precautions and Specific Situations Encountered during Ureteroscopic Lithotripsy

All patients should undergo dipstick and urinary sediment tests, as well as urine culture. If a febrile infection and obstruction are present, drainage with a JJ-stent or percutaneous nephrostomy should be performed before starting active intervention. Urinary infections have to be treated based on the urine culture prior to intervention.

Patients who are receiving anticoagulation agents should be referred to their responsible specialist. If the medication has to be continued or bleeding diathesis cannot be corrected, all treatments except ureteroscopy are contraindicated. Ureteroscopic lithotripsy under general anesthesia is a recommended option in such cases.

Obesity may increase the overall morbidity. The success rate of SWL and PCNL, which are dependent on the techniques used, may be negatively impacted, while ureteroscopy has proven to be effective without being influenced by the body mass index.

Stones composed of calcium oxalate monohydrate, brushite and homogenous cysteine are particularly hard and respond poorly to SWL. Therefore, endourology is preferred if the stone composition is known. Determination of the radiopacity on KUB or measurement of the Hounsfield units on CT scan can be helpful.

Steinstrasse is a frequently encountered obstructing accumulation of stone fragments or stone gravel in the ureter, and occurs in 4-7% of cases after SWL [31]. The stone size is a major factor associated with its formation. When the steinstrasse is not symptomatic, conservative treatment can be the initial treatment option if the patient agrees with a close follow-up schedule. Medical expulsive therapy significantly increases the stone expulsion rate and reduces the need for endoscopic intervention [32]. If spontaneous passage is unlikely, further treatment of the steinstrasse is indicated. SWL treatment is indicated for large stone fragments when a urinary tract infection has been excluded. Ureteroscopy has equal overall efficacy, but complete stone removal is usually achieved after a single treatment [33]. In symptomatic patients where the steinstrasse cannot be passed to allow placement of a JJ-stent, a percutaneous nephrostomy is indicated.

Finally, SWL is contraindicated in pregnant patients. In these cases, conservative management with the placement of a ureteral JJ-stent until the delivery or active removal of stones with URS is generally appropriate.

Conclusion

As technological advances continue to arise throughout the field of endourology, the indications for ureteroscopic lithotripsy continue to change. The guidelines may fall behind the times in just a few years. Surgeons should pursue the development of their own skills and select the most appropriate treatment option for each individual patient based on their skills and experiences.

References

[1] Preminger GM, Tiselius HG, Assimos DG, et al. Guideline for the management of ureteral calculi. *Eur. Urol.* 2007, 52: 1610-31.
[2] Miller OF, Kane CJ. Time to stone passage for observed ureteral calculi: a guide for patient education. *J. Urol.* 1999; 162: 688-90.
[3] Glowacki LS, Beecroft ML, Cook RJ, et al. The natural history of asymptomatic urolithiasis. *J. Urol.* 1992; 147: 319-21.
[4] Burgher A, Beman M, Holtzman JL, et al. Progression of nephrolithiasis: long-term outcomes with observation of asymptomatic calculi. *J. Endourol.* 2004; 18: 534-9.
[5] Hubner W, Porpaczy P. Treatment of calyceal calculi. *Br. J. Urol.* 1990; 66: 9-11.

[6] Inci K, Sahin A, Islamoglu E, et al. Prospective long-term followup of patients with asymptomatic lower pole calyceal stones. *J. Urol.* 2007; 177: 2189-92.
[7] Keely FX Jr, Tilling K, Elves A, et al. Preliminary results of a randomized controlled trial of prophylactic shock wave lithotripsy for small asymptomatic renal calyceal stones. *BJU. Int.* 2001; 87: 1-8.
[8] Collins JW, Keeley FX. Is there a role for prophylactic shock wave lithotripsy for asymptomatic calyceal stones? *Curr. Opin. Urol.* 12: 281−286, 2002.
[9] European Association of Urology (EAU) Guidelines. Guidelines on urolithiasis. EAU 2013.
[10] Scoffone CM, Cracco CM, Cossu M, et al. Endoscopic combined intrarenal surgery in Galdakao-modified supine Valdivia position: a new standard for percutaneous nephrolithotomy? *Eur. Urol.* 2008; 54: 1393-403.
[11] Landman J, Venkatesh R, Lee DI, et al. Combined percutaneous and retrograde approach to staghorn calculi with application of the ureteral access sheath to facilitate percutaneous nephrolithotomy. *J. Urol.* 2003; 169: 64-7.
[12] Breda A, Ogunyemi O, Leppert JT, et al. Flexible ureteroscopy and laser lithotripsy for single intrarenal stone 2 cm or greater – is this the new frontier? *J. Urol.* 2008; 179: 981-4.
[13] Riley JM, Stearman L, Troxel S. Retrograde ureteroscopy for renal stones larger than 2.5 cm. *J. Endourol.* 2009; 23: 1395-8.
[14] Hyams ES, Munver R, Bird VG, et al. Flexible ureteroscopy and holmium laser lithotripsy for the management of renal stone burdens that measure 2 to 3 cm: a multi-institutional experience. *J. Endourol.* 2010; 24: 1583-8.
[15] Takazawa R, Kitayama S, Tsujii T. Successful outcome of flexible ureteroscopy with holmium laser lithotripsy for renal stone 2 cm or greater. *Int. J. Urol.* 2012; 19: 264-7.
[16] Argyropoulos AN, Tolley DA. Evaluation of outcome following lithotripsy. *Curr. Opin. Urol.* 2010; 20: 154-8.
[17] Srisubat A, Potisat S, Lojanapiwat B, et al. Extracorporeal shock wave lithotripsy (ESWL) versus percutaneous nephrolithotomy (PCNL) or retrograde intrarenal surgery (RIRS) for kidney stones. *Cochrane Database Syst. Rev.* 2009; CD007044.
[18] Sahinkanat T, Ekerbicer H, Onal B, et al. Evaluation of the effects of relationships between main spatial lower pole calyceal anatomic factors

on the success of shock-wave lithotripsy in patients with lower pole kidney stones. *Urology.* 2008; 71: 801-5.

[19] Danuser H, Muller R, Descoeudres B, et al. Extracorporeal shock wave lithotripsy of lower calyx calculi: how much is treatment outcome influenced by the anatomy of the collecting system? *Eur. Urol.* 2007; 52: 539-46.

[20] Preminger GM. Management of lower pole renal calculi: shock wave lithotripsy versus percutaneous nephrolithotomy versus flexible ureteroscopy. *Urol. Res.* 2006; 34: 108-11.

[21] Pearle MS, Lingeman JE, Leveillee R, et al. Prospective, randomized trial comparing shock wave lithotripsy and ureteroscopy for lower pole caliceal calculi 1 cm or less. *J. Urol.* 2005; 173: 2005-9.

[22] Manikandan R, Gall Z, Gunendran T, et al. Do anatomic factors pose a significant risk in the formation of lower pole stones? *Urology.* 2007; 69: 620-4.

[23] Juan YS, Chuang SM, Wu WJ, et al. Impact of lower pole anatomy on stone clearance after shock wave lithotripsy. *Kaohsiung. J. Med. Sci.* 2005; 21: 358-64.

[24] Ruggera L, Beltrami P, Ballario R, et al. Impact of anatomical pielocaliceal topography in the treatment of renal lower calyces stones with extracorporeal shock wave lithotripsy. *Int. J. Urol.* 2005; 12: 525-32.

[25] Knoll T, Musial A, Trojan L, et al. Measurement of renal anatomy for prediction of lower-pole calyceal stone clearance: reproducibility of different parameters. *J. Endourol.* 2003; 17: 447.

[26] Sumino Y, Mimata H, Tasaki Y, et al. Predictors of lower pole renal stone clearance after extracorporeal shock wave lithotripsy. *J. Urol.* 2002; 168: 1344-7.

[27] Madbouly K, Sheir KZ, Elsobky E. Impact of lower pole renal anatomy on stone clearance after shock wave lithotripsy: fact or fiction? *J. Urol.* 2001; 165: 1415-8.

[28] Desai M, Ganpule A, Manohar T. "Multiperc" for complete staghorn calculus. *J. Endourol.* 2008; 22: 1831-3.

[29] Akman T, Sari E, Binbay M, et al. Comparison of outcomes after percutaneous nephrolithotomy of staghorn calculi in those with single and multiple accesses. *J. Endourol.* 2010; 24: 955-60.

[30] Geavlete P, Georgescu D, Niță G, et al. Complications of 2735 retrograde semirigid ureteroscopy procedures: a single-center experience. *J. Endourol.* 2006; 20: 179-85.

[31] Sayed MA, el-Taher AM, Aboul-Ella HA, et al. Steinstrasse after extracorporeal shockwave lithotripsy: aetiology, prevention and management. *BJU. Int.* 2001; 88: 675-8.

[32] Resim S, Ekerbicer HC, Ciftci A, et al. Role of tamsulosin in treatment of patients with steinstrasse developing after shock wave lithotripsy. *Urology.* 2005; 66: 945-8.

[33] Rabbani SM. Treatment of steinstrasse by transureteral lithotripsy. *Urol. J.* 2008; 5: 89-93.

PART II. INSTRUMENTATION

Chapter 2

Instrumentation for Ureteroscopic Lithotripsy

Ryoji Takazawa[*], *M.D., Ph.D., Sachi Kitayama, M.D.*
and Toshihiko Tsujii, M.D., Ph.D.

Department of Urology, Tokyo Metropolitan Ohtsuka Hospital,
Tokyo, Japan

Abstract

A thorough working knowledge of the various ureteroscopes and associated endoscopic instruments currently available is crucial to the successful treatment of urinary calculi. In this chapter, the instrumentation currently available for ureteroscopic lithotripsy is discussed. The system of ureteroscopes has developed from rod-lens systems to fiberoptic systems, and now digital optical systems. The guidewires differ with respect to size, tip design, rigidity, flexibility and coating material. Ureteral access sheaths are now available in various sizes. A good irrigation system is crucial to successful treatment. Knowledge about the properties of the holmium:YAG laser is important to perform successful operations. Understanding the history of the development of stone baskets is also helpful for good performance.

---

[*] Corresponding author: Ryoji Takazawa, M.D., Ph.D. ryoji_takazawa@tmhp.jp.

Ureteral stents have been available in various sizes, but the indication for their placement after ureteroscopic lithotripsy is still under discussion.

Introduction

A thorough working knowledge of the various ureteroscopes and associated endoscopic instruments currently available is crucial to the successful treatment of urinary calculi. The following ureteroscopic equipment will be discussed in detail in this chapter.

1. Ureteroscopes
2. Guidewires
3. Ureteral access sheaths
4. Irrigation systems
5. The holmium:YAG laser
6. Stone baskets
7. Ureteral stents

1. Ureteroscopes

The goal of endoscopy is to access and treat organs, through natural or artificial orifices in the body, with a telescoping device. The gradual evolution toward the modern endoscopes began with Philipp Bozzini's construction of the "lichtleiter" in 1806 for direct inspection and treatment of the uterus and bladder. These early endoscopes were cumbersome and impractical, made of hollow examining tubes with illumination provided by candle light directed by a mirror. With the advances in materials science and optics, endoscopes have undergone major refinements since Bozzini's lichtleiter.

1.1. History

In 1912, Young and Mckay performed the first ureteroscopic procedure using a 9.5 Fr pediatric cystoscope in a two-month-old child with a posterior urethral valve [1]. It is from this initial experience that ureteroscopy began its long evolutionary course. Our modern day concept of endoscopy of the ureter and renal pelvis was first made possible by Marshall in 1960 with the advent of a 3-mm flexible fiberscope [2]. Marshall visualized a ureteral calculus with a fiber-optic bundled catheter. In 1977, Goodman passed an 11 Fr pediatric cystoscope into the ureter and fulgurated a low grade urothelial carcinoma of the ureter [3]. In 1978, Lyon dilated the distal ureter to 16 Fr with Jewett sounds in order to perform ureteroscopy with a 14 Fr resectoscope [4]. The first practical ureteroscopes were developed in 1980 and 1981 by Enrique Perez-Castro and the Karl Storz Company, respectively [5]. However, these ureteroscopes utilized the rod-lens optical system and were limited by their size and the lack of adequate instrumentation for stone fragmentation and removal. They were purely instruments for diagnosis, and were not practical for therapeutic use.

The application of fiberoptic technology was the next major step in the development of ureteroscopes. This was based on the principle of total internal reflection; light traveling inside of an ultrathin glass fiber surrounded by a cladding with a lower refractory index can be transmitted over a long distance with minimal degradation. A coherent fiberoptic bundle contains thousands of individual fibers with identical orientation at the end of each bundle, thus, the exact image is transmitted to the eyepiece. Therefore, the image obtained by fiberoptic bundles is not a single image, but a composite matrix of each fiber within the bundle, giving it a "honeycomb" appearance.

The early flexible ureteroscopes were limited by the lack of irrigation, active deflection and/or instrumentation. In 1968, Takayasu and Aso developed the first flexible ureterorenoscope with an operating channel [6]. Continuous refinements have led to today's flexible ureteroscopes with high pixel densities. These ureteroscopes contain two coherent bundles for light transmission and one noncoherent bundle for image transmission, a working/irrigation channel to allow for both irrigation and insertion of instruments, and active dual deflection, as well as secondary passive deflection.

As the demand for reliable rigid ureteroscopes grew, the fiberoptic technology was applied to a new generation of "semirigid" fiberoptic ureteroscopes. The flexibility of the fiberoptic bundles allowed for the metal shaft to be flexed up to two inches off the vertical axis without significant image distortion. It also allowed a significant reduction of the outside diameter of the endoscopes, while maintaining larger working channels and a greater irrigation flow rate compared to "rigid" ureteroscopes with the rod-lens system.

1.2. Semirigid Ureteroscopes

The newer generation semirigid ureteroscopes contain fiberoptic bundles larger than those in a flexible ureteroscope. Therefore, the image is comparable to those derived from a rod-lens system, and the "honeycomb" effect is further reduced by new fiber-packing techniques and advanced camera systems. Semirigid ureteroscopes are currently available in many designs, as shown in Table 1.

Semirigid ureteroscopes have the advantage of providing good image transmission and larger working channels. Most of the semirigid ureteroscopes have a round or oval tip, designed to reduce trauma to both the ureter and to the ureteral orifice while introducing the ureteroscope. The shaft design is commonly triangular or oval. The shafts of these scopes are tapered such that they gradually enlarge from 6-8 Fr at the distal tip to 8-10 Fr at the proximal shaft. This design increases the proximal strength of the scope while providing a gradual dilation of the ureter as the instrument is advanced.

The working channel is an important feature which allows for simultaneous instrument passage and irrigation. The inclusion of a single, straight, large working channel is possible in ureteroscopes with an offset eyepiece. In contrast, two channel scopes allow for the passage of a working instrument without a diminution in the flow of irrigation. These scopes usually have a 4 Fr working channel that can accommodate a standard 3 Fr instrument and a 2 Fr irrigation channel. The smallest diameter ureteroscope that will allow for adequate visualization and treatment should be selected.

1.3. Flexible Ureteroscopes

The tortuosity of the ureter proximal to the iliac vessels makes semirigid ureteroscopy more difficult in this region. Flexible ureteroscopes offer the ability to better navigate the upper ureter and renal pelvis, and their development has improved the ability to treat ureteral calculi. The flexible ureteroscope can more effectively reach all areas of the urinary tract.

Like the semirigid ureteroscopes, the tip of the flexible ureteroscope is commonly beveled to protect against ureteral injury. The distal tip size of flexible ureteroscopes ranges from 5 to 9 Fr. The flexible ureteroscope can be actively deflected. The tip deflection angle has improved with technological advances, with newer ureteroscopes able to offer 270 deflection capabilities in both the upward and downward directions. The smaller size and greater flexibility of the laser probes, in conjunction with flexible ureteroscopes, offer the ability to access and treat urinary calculi in almost all locations. The 200 micron laser fiber and nitinol-based baskets that are currently available have only a minimal influence on the deflection capabilities of flexible ureteroscopes.

The common working paradigms for the available fiberoptic flexible ureteroscopes are fairly similar, although different manufacturers may point out unique manufacturer-specific features and variations in basic construct. In general, the ureteroscope consists of a handle with an eyepiece and a long flexible shaft. The shaft contains both fibers for transmission of the images and for the transmission of light. The arrangement of bundles in ureteroscopes from different manufacturers varies slightly in this respect. The fibers transmit the images to the more proximally located lens and eyepiece. Deflection is accomplished by means of a lever/pulley mechanism that may operate with either intuitive or counterintuitive deflection. The handle also includes ports of variable configuration that allow for working elements to be passed down a channel that travels through the shaft to the tip. This same mechanism allows for irrigation to pass in a similar manner. For this reason, as is well known to many users, the irrigation flow may be increased or decreased to variable degrees depending on what working elements are being passed through the working channel.

A number of fiberoptic flexible ureteroscopes from a variety of manufacturers are available for use. These ureteroscopes are summarized in Table 2, along with a number of commonly noted parameters, including the caliber along their shaft, degree and direction of deflection, working length and diameter of working channels.

The Gyrus ACMI (now a business division of Olympus) DUR 8 Elite ureteroscope has two points of active deflection, accomplished by use of a second lever that provides deflection of the scope more proximal on the shaft. The active secondary deflection adds 130 degrees down. This scope has also been equipped with a moiré reduction filter. Moiré patterns are often an undesired artifact of images produced by various imaging techniques. The DUR 8 Ultra has been created as a successor to the DUR 8 Elite. This ureteroscope is a hybrid of Olympus and ACMI technologies. The ureteroscope has been enhanced so that it has 270 degrees of up and down deflection.

The Olympus URF-P5 is an enhanced version of the prior Olympus fiberoptic flexible ureteroscopes URF-P3. This ureteroscope has a 5.3 Fr bullet-shaped tip. This scope has an incorporated moiré reduction filter to enhance images and provide a clearer picture. The deflective portion of the shaft is covered with thicker rubber to resist potential puncturing. The Olympus URF-P6 is the newest fiberoptic flexible ureteroscope. This new ureteroscope has a smaller tip diameter (4.9 Fr) and a smaller shaft diameter (7.95 Fr), while it has the same working channel size (3.6 Fr) and dual 270 degrees of up and down deflection.

The Storz Flex X2 ureteroscope is similar to its predecessor, the Flex X scope, in many respects. Due to general concerns regarding laser damage caused by all flexible ureteroscopes, this ureteroscope was enhanced with the addition of a new material, laserite^{TM}, at its distal tip, in an attempt to make this portion of the ureteroscope more resistant to potential laser-induced damage.

Richard Wolf produces the Viper and a more advanced flexible ureteroscope, the Cobra, which features dual channels for the simultaneous use of two devices, such as a laser and basket. The dual 3.3 Fr channels accommodate continuous irrigation capabilities with increased flow. The Cobra also includes an ergonomic laser dial with an integrated locking mechanism to advance the laser fiber and minimize laser damage.

1.4. Digital Ureteroscopes

Beyond doubt, the introduction of fiberoptic flexible ureteroscopes revolutionized urological practice for the management of upper urinary tract pathologies. Nonetheless, despite widespread of use with these ureteroscopes, a number of concerns persist. Fiberoptic ureteroscopes tend to produce a grainy image, water may leak into the lens, and fibers may burn out and fracture, resulting in a loss of image quality. The images produced by fiberoptic flexible ureteroscopes are not as sharp as those from semirigid ureteroscopes due to the smaller number of pixels in the flexible instrument's image. The image quality may be improved by increasing the diameter of the flexible ureteroscope, but this is likely to increase the risk of failure of access to the upper urinary tract and lead to decreased flexibility. Therefore, a strong impetus was present for improvement of the available flexible ureteroscopes.

The key paradigm change with regard to digital flexible ureteroscopes was the "chip on tip" design, where an image is picked up, at times processed, transmitted by a digital sensor and sent to a proximal point via a single wire, where further processing and transmission take place. This arrangement bypasses the fragile optical fiber system of conventional fiberoptic flexible ureteroscopes. This arrangement may also include a more luminous distal light source built into the ureteroscope itself.

The specific configuration and operative paradigm of the available digital ureteroscopes vary in certain aspects. The Gyrus ACMI DUR D and Storz Flex XC flexible ureteroscopes have distally located light-emitting diode (LED) light sources and a distally located complementary metal oxide semiconductor (CMOS) chip that picks up and processes images. The Olympus digital ureteroscope, URF-V, has a light source that is transmitted from a proximal source and a charge-coupled device (CCD) chip that picks up images and transmits the data to a proximal source for processing. At the current time, it is of unknown significance what these different arrangements will mean for long-term scope operation, durability and the chance for malfunction or catastrophic failure.

The digital ureteroscopes which are now available for use can be seen in Table 3. Due to design changes, the digital ureteroscopes are all lighter than their fiberoptic counterparts. All digital ureteroscopes provide high-quality digital images, autofocusing capabilities and digital magnification, which improve the user experience. The overall experience with digital ureteroscopes is growing, but is still somewhat limited.

The Gyrus ACMI Invisio DUR D was the first digital flexible ureteroscope. The format of the hand piece, deflective mechanism, working port and channels is relatively similar to its fiberoptic counterparts. The tip of the scope contains the dual LED light carriers and a 1-mm digital camera. The LED light can last for up to 10,000 hours, which is significantly longer than more expensive xenon light sources. The ureteroscope has a configuration such that it is simply plugged in and ready for use. Of interest, the two aforementioned technological advances significantly reduced the weight of the scope (DUR D 505 g vs. DUR 8E 1012 g). The internalization of the light source also reduces the risks of burning or fires. This ureteroscope also has a laser fiber detection system (IDC-1500-endoscope protection system) which can detect when the blue coating of a laser fiber is retracted within the ureteroscope, and alerts the operator. This option can be used to automatically disable (place on standby) the laser generator, with the goal of preventing laser-induced ureteroscope damage.

An Olympus digital flexible ureteroscope, the URF-V, is also available and currently in use. This digital ureteroscope contains a CCD chip and has light transmitted from a proximal source. This scope is also fitted with moiré reduction capability.

Table 1. The semirigid ureteroscopes

Manufacturer	Model	Working length (cm)	Tip size (Fr)	Mid-shaft size (Fr)	Proximal shaft size (Fr)	Channel size (Fr)
Olympus-Gyrus ACMI	MR-6LA MR-6A	41 33	6.9	-	-	3.4 & 2.3
Olympus	WA29040A WA29041A	43 33	6.4	7.8	-	4.2
Olympus	WA29042A	43	8.6	9.8	-	6.4
Olympus	WA29043A	43	7.5	7.5	-	3.4 & 2.4
Storz	27001 L 27001 K	43 34	7.0	-	13.5	5.0
Storz	27002 L 27002 K	43 34	7.0	-	13.5	6.0
Storz	27010 L 27010 K	43 34	7.0	8.4	9.9	3.4 & 2.4
EMS	FR107	43	8	-	9.8	5.3
EMS	FR108	43	6	-	7.5	4.1
Wolf	8708.534	43	6.5	-	8.5	4 &2.4 (dual working channel)

Table 2. The fiberoptic flexible ureteroscopes

Manufacturer	Model	Working length (cm)	Tip size (Fr)	Mid-shaft size (Fr)	Deflection up/down (degrees)	Channel size (Fr)
Olympus-Gyrus ACMI	DUR 8 Elite	64	6.8	8.7	170/180+130	3.6
Olympus-Gyrus ACMI	DUR 8 Ultra	67	6.8	8.7	270/270	3.6
Olympus	URF-P5	70	5.3	8.4	180/275	3.6
Olympus	URF-P6	67	4.9	7.95	275/275	3.6
Storz	Flex X2	67	7.5	8.4	270/270	3.6
Wolf	Viper	68	6.0	8.8	270/270	3.6
Wolf	Cobra	68	6.0	9.9	270/270	3.3/3.3 (dual working channel)

Table 3. The digital flexible ureteroscopes

Manufacturer	Model	Working length (cm)	Tip size (Fr)	Mid-shaft size (Fr)	Maximum shaft size (Fr)	Deflection up/down (degrees)	Channel size (Fr)	Light source/chip
Olympus-Gyrus ACMI	Invisio DUR D	65	8.7	-	-	250/250	3.6	LED/CMOS
Olympus	URF-V	67	8.5	9.9	10.8	180/275	3.6	Fiber/CCD
Storz	Flex XC	70	8.5	8.5	-	270/270	3.6	LED/CMOS

In addition, this ureteroscope has narrow band imaging (NBI) capability, which operates by alteration of the white light source to specific wavelength bands, which is useful for observing the mucosal morphology. This modality is currently being used in a number of settings.

The Storz FLEX XC has also recently become available for use. This digital ureteroscope has a design similar to that of the DUR D in that it contains LED and CMOS technology. A notable difference in this digital ureteroscope is that it retains a relatively small caliber shaft along its working length. The FLEX XC, like its most recent fiberoptic counterpart, is equipped with laserite^{TM}.

2. Guidewires

Guidewires are used to gain access to the ureter, which is the initial step in most ureteroscopic surgeries. The guidewires differ with respect to size, tip design, rigidity, flexibility and the coating material. Knowledge of these basic properties is essential when choosing the correct wire for a particular clinical situation. The ideal guidewire should be flexible enough to bypass any point of obstruction, firm enough to secure access in the desired kidney, rigid enough to permit the passage of instruments and soft enough to do all of the above without traumatizing the urinary tract.

2.1. History

Guidewires were initially developed for vascular access and passage of intraluminal devices. In the technique attributed to Dr. Sven-Ivar Seldinger, the desired vessel is punctured with a hollow needle, a guidewire is passed through the needle, the needle is withdrawn, a blunt-tipped catheter or other endovascular instrument is passed into the vessel lumen over the wire, and finally, the wire is withdrawn once access is secured [7]. Similarly, guidewires were adopted in urologic practice in 1981 to address anatomical and situational difficulties that prevented retrograde ureteral intubation with standard catheters [8]. Guidewires have since become a standard tool in the endourologist's armamentarium for use in routine stent placement and flexible and semirigid ureteroscopy. Moreover, they have become essential in the completion of complex cases, including those with tortuous ureters, heterotopic orifices and impacted stones. A variety of guidewires exist, and knowledge of four basic properties of guidewires is essential for choosing the correct wire for a particular clinical situation: the size, tip design, rigidity and surface coating.

2.2. Size

Typically, the wire diameter ranges from 0.018 to 0.038 inches. The guidewire length ranges from 145 to 260 cm. Although individual preferences vary, we generally use a 150 cm, 0.035 inch, guidewire for standard ureteroscopic procedures. Wires shorter than this may make it more difficult to pass a flexible ureteroscope, while longer wires are simply unnecessary and can become entangled or accidentally pulled from outside the patient, resulting in lost access.

2.3. Tip Design

Wire tips are available in straight, angled and J-types. Straight-tipped wires are most commonly used for routine ureteroscopy. Most wires used in current practice lead with a soft, floppy tip designed to prevent iatrogenic ureteral or renal trauma. These flexible tips are available in a standard length of 3 cm. Angled-tipped wires are often utilized for accessing laterally displaced orifices or navigating beyond points of obstruction or tortuosity. J-tipped wires are most commonly used to establish access within a calyx during percutaneous nephrolithotomy. In order to facilitate passage into an infundibulum or the ureteropelvic junction, the J-tip can be applied, allowing increased tension to be placed on the outer core of the wire.

2.4. Rigidity

Urological guidewire shafts are composed of a solid metal core surrounded by a steel outer coil. The core is made of either steel or nitinol, a metal alloy made of nickel and titanium that allows for shape memory and super-elasticity, while providing columnar strength to resist kinking. An increased shaft stiffness is useful for straightening tortuous ureters and serving as a working wire in cases where a routine guidewire is inadequate. The wire core is tapered as it approaches the tip, and the length and degree of tapering determine the tip flexibility.

2.5. Surface Coating

Guidewire surfaces are generally coated with polytetrafluoroethylene (PTFE) or hydrophilic materials, both of which are designed to create a frictionless surface. We prefer to use PTFE-coated wires because they are easier to handle. If a PTFE-coated guidewire cannot pass through a tight stricture or impacted stones, hydrophilic guidewires may overcome the difficulty. These wires can become quite slippery due to their hydrophilic nature, and thus should not be utilized as a safety wire. They may become displaced more easily and compromise the ureteral access. If access is achieved with a hydrophilic guidewire, it should be exchanged, if possible, for a PTFE-coated wire in order to prevent loss of access. A torque device can be used with hydrophilic wires for added control and assistance with maneuvering the wire into its desired position. Dry gauze can be wrapped around the wire and manipulated by the surgeon to achieve the same result.

3. Ureteral Access Sheaths

The ureteral access sheath (UAS), first introduced by Takayasu and Aso in 1974, has proven to be a useful adjunct in ureteroscopy [9]. Routine use of a UAS is recommended in flexible ureteroscopic procedures. In addition to easy re-entry to the ureter, UAS have been shown to decrease the intrarenal pressure while significantly increasing the irrigation flow, and also to minimize the ureteral trauma associated with repeated passage of the ureteroscope during withdrawal of stone fragments. Due to these characteristics, a UAS may provide surgeons with better visualization during ureteroscopic stone extraction, as well as decreasing the risk of complications.

3.1. Procedures

Current ureteral access sheaths consist of an outer sheath and a tapered dilating obturator. They are frequently coated with hydrophilic polymers designed to decrease friction during passage, allowing for easier insertion. An inner dilator with a tapered distal end provides a mechanical dilating force to aid in sheath advancement. UAS are sized based on both the inner and outer diameters of the sheath. Recently, various sheaths sizes and lengths have become available, as shown in Table 4. The most common size and length is 12/14 Fr and 35 cm.

Prior to UAS deployment, a 0.035-inch stiff guidewire is placed in the upper tract under fluoroscopic guidance. The UAS is then moistened to ensure lubrication, and is advanced over the stiff wire to a level just below the ureteral calculus under fluoroscopic guidance. When used with flexible ureteroscopy in the kidney, the sheath can be positioned at or just below the ureteropelvic junction. Once the access sheath is advanced to the proper level, the inner dilator and working wire are removed, and the ureteroscope is inserted into the sheath for subsequent stone fragmentation and removal.

While a UAS may be used in the majority of cases using a flexible ureteroscope, it is not uncommon to encounter difficulty in passing the UAS. We found that young patients and the patients with duplicated collecting systems usually have small caliber ureters. If UAS placement is difficult, gentle coaxial dilation with the internal obturator of the UAS may prove useful. However, care should be taken to avoid applying excess sheer force that could lead to ureteral injury or avulsion. If this procedure fails, we place an indwelling ureteral JJ-stent, which allows for passive ureteral dilation and successful UAS or ureteroscope insertion in seven to 10 days. We generally avoid balloon dilation in order to decrease the risk of ureteral injury by aggressive dilation.

3.2. Stone-Free Rates

Surgeons have postulated that UASs improve the stone-free rates following ureteroscopy by allowing for passive irrigation of stone fragments, as well as quicker access to the upper collecting system. Previously published reports have listed stone-free rates with the use of a UAS ranging from 77-86% [10, 11], while the rates without the use of a UAS ranged from 72-84% [12-16].

L'Esperance et al. have published the only study directly evaluating the effect of UAS utilization on the stone-free rates following ureteroscopy.

Table 4. The commonly available ureteral access sheaths

Manufacturer	Product name	Size, inner/outer (Fr)	Length (cm)
Cook	Flexor	9.5/11.5, 12/14, 14/16	13, 20, 28, 35, 45, 55
BARD	Aqua Guide	10/12, 10/14, 11/13, 11/15	25, 35, 45, 55
Boston Scientific	Navigator	11/13, 12/14, 13/15	28, 36, 46
Coloplast-Porges	Retrace	10/12, 12/14	35, 45

Following a retrospective review of their clinical database, they identified a total of a 256 ureteroscopic procedures performed for renal calculi, 173 of which were performed with the use of a UAS. The demographic data, stone burden and stone location were similar between the groups. The authors found that the overall stone-free rates were significantly improved in the patients in whom a UAS was utilized 79% vs. 67%, p=0.042 [17].

3.3. Increased Renal Pressure

Increased intrarenal pressure has long been a concern during ureteroscopy. Attempts to maintain good visualization may inadvertently raise the intrarenal pressure and over-distend the renal pelvis, resulting in pyelosinus/pyelovenous backflow. The adverse effects of increased renal pelvic pressure have been documented in animal studies [18]. At pressures exceeding 150 mmHg, many pathological changes begin to occur. These include submucosal edema, vasculitis, tubular vacuolization and focal renal scarring. As the pressures rise above 330 mmHg, rupture of the collecting system can occur. These are all real risks in the modern era of ureteroscopy with hand irrigation, where pressures can exceed 400 mmHg.

The ability of the UAS to lower the renal pressure has been demonstrated in several well-designed studies. Functioning as an open conduit into the kidney, it allows fluid to enter through the endoscope, and to flow out through the sheath around the scope, thereby decreasing the renal pelvic pressure. Landman et al. demonstrated this relationship using the *en bloc* urinary tract from cadaveric donors [19]. In their study, lower pole percutaneous access with a 30 Fr sheath was gained into the kidney, and a nephroscope was then advanced into the renal pelvis. Irrigation was infused through the nephroscope at varying rates, while the intrarenal pressure and irrigation flow rates were measured under a variety of ureteral drainage conditions. The modes of ureteral drainage included the native ureter, a 6 Fr ureteral catheter, a 10/12 Fr 35cm UAS, 12/14 Fr 35cm UAS and a 7 Fr occlusion balloon catheter. Importantly, the intrarenal pressures were significantly lower while using both the 10/12 Fr and 12/14 Fr UASs compared to the other conditions.

Ureteral access sheaths have also been shown to decrease the renal pelvic pressure during ureteroscopy in a cadaveric model. Using a percutaneous pressure monitor, Rehman et al. were able to record the renal pelvic pressure while performing ureteroscopy with a 7.5 Fr flexible ureteroscope [20]. The ureteroscopes were then introduced into the collecting system using a 35 cm

UAS with varying diameters (10/12 Fr, 12/14 Fr and 14/16 Fr) or were introduced unsheathed (control). The author then delivered irrigation through the ureteroscope at pressures of 50, 100 or 200 mmHg while measuring intrarenal pressure and irrigation flow. The irrigation flow was higher in all of the UASs tested compared to the control. In all experimental conditions with a UAS in place, the intrarenal pressure was noted to stay below 30 cm H_2O. Notably, at low irrigation pressures (50 cmH_2O), the flow through each sheath was similar, but at increasing pressures, the 12/14 Fr and 14/16 Fr sheaths had better pressure and flow characteristics than the 10/12 Fr sheath. The authors also noted that the 12/14 Fr sheath performed equally well as the 14/16 Fr sheath, and concluded that the 12/14 Fr UAS optimizes the pressure and flow characteristics while limiting the UAS diameter.

3.4. Length of the Procedure

By simplifying repeated access to the upper urinary tract, the UAS has proven beneficial in reducing the time and cost associated with procedure. To study these issues, Kourambas et al. prospectively analyzed a cohort of 59 patients presenting for endoscopy above the level of the iliac vessels [10]. The patients were randomized to ureteroscopy with or without the use of a UAS. The authors utilized a 12/14 Fr hydrophilic coated UAS ranging from 20 to 35 cm depending on the patient size, sex and stone location. They found that the length of the operation was significantly shorter in the patients randomized to the use of a UAS (43 min vs. 53 min, $p<0.05$). Despite having a higher total stone burden in these patients (13.7 mm vs. 10.1 mm, respectively), the stone-free rates between these two groups were similar.

3.5. Decreased Ureteral Blood Flow and Ureteral Strictures

Concerns about ureteral ischemia and eventual ureteral stricture following UAS utilization have been raised. Lullas et al. evaluated this question in a porcine model by measuring the ureteral blood flow at five-minute intervals both with and without a UAS in place [21]. In all study groups, the ureteral blood flow decreased upon UAS insertion. The nadir blood flow was measured at 25% below baseline for the 10/12 Fr sheath, and at 65% below baseline with the 12/14 Fr and 14/16 Fr sheaths. However, this decrease in perfusion was only transient, with ureteral blood flow tending toward normal by 70 minutes;

to 88%, 70% and 68% of the baseline, respectively. However, it should be noted that the 14/16 Fr sheath did reach the nadir level fastest, and also took the longest to normalize after removal of the UAS.

The authors then performed a histological analysis on the ureters from the study. Ureteral specimens were collected at three time points: (1) immediately after the procedure, (2) 48 hours post-procedure and (3) 72 hours post-procedure. At the longer time points, the access sheath group demonstrated nuclear changes, inflammation and increased deposition of collagen, leading to thickening of the ureteral wall, but importantly, no overt signs of ischemic necrosis were evident. While some investigators may argue that these changes could lead to an increased risk of ureteral stricture, this has never proven to be true in a well-designed study.

While evidence from randomized trials is generally lacking, multiple studies have suggested various benefits of UAS use. The decreased length of the operation, reduction in ureteroscope damage and improvement in the stone-free rates all appear to be benefits of using a UAS. This tool will therefore likely remain an important part of the urologist's armamentarium.

4. Irrigation Systems

Historically, natural antegrade urine flow was the primary source of irrigation for urinary endoscopy. With the development of the working channel of the endoscope, the use of active retrograde fluid irrigation has drastically improved upper urinary collecting system endoscopy [6].

4.1. Irrigation Systems

To date, the irrigation systems vary from gravity dependent systems to those operated by repetitive hand or foot control. The gravity-based irrigation systems create the least amount of pressure (50 mmHg), but the pressure cannot be controlled by the surgeon, and may occasionally result in an impaired visual field. Pressure bags can be placed around the irrigation fluid to augment the irrigation flow, and this can be titrated by the surgeon using the stopcock on the endoscope. In contrast, hand and foot pump irrigation systems are actively controlled by the surgeon, resulting in peaks of high flow and pressure (up to 410 mmHg) according to the energy dispended onto the pump.

Using a hand-held irrigation system device is recommended during retrograde ureteroscopy for its capacity to clear the visual field and also for providing a meticulous manual regulation of the flow intensity when demanded by the surgeon. Moreover, it is worth noting that several important factors affect the success of the irrigation techniques, including the use of a ureteral access sheath, the size of the working channel, the tip deflection in flexible ureteroscopes; the number, size and composition of the instruments placed in the working channel; and of course, the type of irrigation system and irrigation fluids used.

4.2. Irrigation Fluids

The irrigation fluid must be transparent, thin, sterile, warm, without debris and chemically innocuous to the human tissue in order to be eligible for use during urinary endoscopy. During a ureteroscopic procedure, fluid flow not only clears away blood, urine and debris from the optical field, but also distends the collecting system, permitting a thorough inspection of endoluminal structures.

Physiological saline encompasses all of the above-mentioned requisites, and it prevents electrolyte imbalance (hyponatremia) in the presence of mild to moderate fluid absorption, as in the case of occasional pyelolymphatic/ pyelovenous backflow during a high-pressure ureteroscopic procedure. However, fluid overload, congestive heart failure, hypothermia and hemolysis are associated with high fluid absorption seen with long operations. Exposure to high intrarenal pressures or serious urothelial rupture with retroperitoneal extravasation may jeopardize not only the endoscopic treatment success, but also the patient's well-being [22, 23]. Given the factual risks of clinically relevant adverse events related to the use of retrograde ureteroscopy, identifying adjunctive measures by which the intrarenal pressure can be lowered may be protective for the patient.

For this reason, the use of pharmacological agents in the irrigation fluid has been postulated, based on the premise that the renal pelvis and ureter have adrenergic, cholinergic and muscarinic receptors that directly interact to affect the endoluminal pressure [24-27]. It has been demonstrated in an *in vivo* study that the use of catecholamines relaxes the ureteral muscle in an animal model. This relaxant effect was attributed to activation of beta 2 and 3 receptors in the ureteral segment immersed in a saline solution with catecholamines [28]. In another animal study, endoluminal norepinephrine injection into the ureter inhibited peristalsis, resulting in a decrease of the smooth muscle tonus, which in turn eliminated the phasic pressure response to perfusion [24]. The most potent relaxing catecholamine was isoproterenol, followed by epinephrine and norepinephrine [26]. These studies suggest that it is possible to obtain a direct local response with regard to the endoluminal pressure by adding one of the above-mentioned catecholamines in the irrigation fluid, and this occurs without systemic adverse events [26-28].

There have been reports on the injection of calcium channel blockers, such as verapamil and theophylline, into the ureter to reduce the smooth muscle peristalsis, and therefore the endoluminal ureteral pressure, with promising results. No side effects were cited and the *in vivo* peristalsis was successfully inhibited [29].

The endoluminal administration of pharmacological agents with the irrigation fluid may, in the near future, be a viable and safe option for reducing the potential hazards of high intrarenal pressures during retrograde urinary tract endoscopy.

5. The Holmium: YAG Laser

The holmium: yttrium-aluminum-garnet (Ho: YAG) laser has dramatically improved intraluminal lithotripsy. After being used initially to treat biliary calculi, the Ho: YAG laser was reported to be a safe and effective method for inducing intracorporeal urinary stone fragmentation in 1995 [30]. Since that initial report, the Ho: YAG laser has become the gold standard for intracorporeal lithotripsy during ureteroscopic procedures. Several properties of this laser have resulted in its widespread adoption.

5.1. The Properties of the Ho: YAG Laser

The Ho: YAG laser has a wavelength of 2,100 nm, which is highly absorbed in 3 mm of water and less than 0.5 mm of tissue, making it ideal for the urological environment. Although the Ho: YAG laser can cause ureteral perforation, it is unlikely to cause significant trauma because of its shallow tissue penetration. The laser energy is transmitted from the laser source efficiently via low OH-silica fibers that are relatively inexpensive and widely available. The fibers may be constructed with small diameters that permit them to be passed through the working channel of both semirigid and flexible endoscopes. The typical fiber core sizes used in ureteroscopy are 365 μm and 200 μm.

The primary mechanism of action of the Ho: YAG laser for lithotripsy is photothermal ablation, although some weak photoacoustic effects also likely occur. The tip of the laser fiber must be brought into direct contact with the stone. Retropulsion during lithotripsy can be problematic, leading to stone migration, but it is reduced with the Ho: YAG laser compared to other types of lasers and pneumatic lithotripsy. The Ho: YAG laser will fragment all types of urinary calculi, including very hard stones. such as cysteine, calcium oxalate monohydrate and calcium phosphate brushite stones.

The Ho: YAG laser allows the user to select the fiber size, the pulse energy and the frequency setting. Our practice is to routinely start with pulse energy and frequency settings of 0.6 J at 6 Hz. If the stone is very hard and not fragmented efficiently, the energy and frequency settings are gradually increased up to 1.0 J at 10 Hz. Increasing the pulse energy above 1.0 J is rarely needed for the treatment of ureteral and renal stones.

The Lumenis VersaPulse 100W laser provides additional flexibility, with a pulse energy setting as low as 0.2 J and a pulse frequency setting as high as 50 Hz. While the lower pulse energy setting may be less efficient with regard to the fragmentation speed, it creates smaller stone fragments and less retropulsion. Coupled with a high pulse frequency setting of 50 Hz, this creates a "dusting" effect of the stone. This may be useful when the surgeon does not want to basket extract pieces, or for larger stones where creating less fragments may be desirable [31].

5.2. Laser Fibers

The laser fibers should be advanced with the flexible endoscope undeflected so as to minimize the risk of trauma to the working channel. Once deployed, they are sufficiently compliant such that there is minimal detriment in the deflection capability, and have demonstrated higher stone-free rates than both pneumatic and electrohydraulic lithotrites. A larger fiber results in a more dramatic reduction in the flow rate through the ureteroscope as compared to a smaller diameter fiber.

Another important aspect of the fiber performance is the ability of the fiber to deflect easily so as to not limit the deflection of the ureteroscope. Studies have demonstrated that, while the 365 um fiber provides better durability and overall stone fragmentation, the 200 um fiber better mitigates the reduction in deflection capability during flexible ureteroscopy. We typically utilize a laser setting of 0.6-0.8 J and 6-8 Hz. We recommend increasing the frequency rather than the energy setting if the stone does not fragment sufficiently. Lower energy settings lead to smaller stone fragments and less degradation of the laser fiber tip.

6. Stone Baskets

Thanks to the development of smaller flexible and semirigid ureteroscopes, the field of endourology has made dramatic improvements. There have been equally dramatic improvements in ureteroscopic instrumentation that have allowed ureteroscopy to become a therapeutic, and not merely diagnostic, modality. In this section, the history of stone baskets will be briefly reviewed, and the currently available stone baskets will be described.

6.1. History

Early in the history of endourology, treatment of small lower ureteral stones was accomplished by blind maneuvering of baskets, followed by manual extraction. With the development of ureteroscopes, the baskets were used under fluoroscopic guidance and direct vision. When the flexible ureteroscope was introduced in the early 1980s, flexible working instruments were developed. The more recently developed instruments can maintain the maximal scope deflection and irrigation flow, while optimizing the performance.

The earliest stone baskets were the Dormia baskets; a classical helical structure that facilitated capture of the stone and subsequent withdrawal. The Dormia baskets were constructed with three or four wires, with or without a filiform tip that could be passed beyond the stone. With the introduction of percutaneous stone removal in the late 1970s, the helical design of the Dormia basket proved unsuitable for use in the kidney, especially for the removal of calyceal stones. The major problem associated with the use of these baskets was trauma to the collecting system from a rigid tip extending beyond the cage, particularly if the stone was in a calyx.

The next generation of baskets included the Segura stainless steel flat-wire basket, which was introduced in the early 1980s. This basket could open widely in a relatively small space, which allowed the capture of stones from the renal pelvis and calyces during percutaneous nephrolithotomy (PCNL). Although the Segura basket rapidly gained popularity, the rigid steel wires limited the deflection of flexible nephroscopes, and the protruding tip limited access to smaller calyces and tended to traumatize the papilla, causing bleeding.

The introduction of the nitinol tipless basket marked the transition to the modern era of endourology [32]. The N-Circle® (Cook) was the first nitinol basket introduced. Nitinol is a combination of nickel and titanium, and the flexibility of the material allowed full deflection of nephroscopes, and later, flexible ureteroscopes. The tipless design and the flexibility of nitinol prevented trauma to the papilla during the removal of calyceal stones. The combination of nitinol and the tipless design enabled the immediate opening of the basket, allowing the capture of stones almost anywhere in the collecting system.

Miniatuarization of tipless nitinol baskets as small as 1.3 Fr in diameter allowed improved irrigation when used with flexible ureteroscopes. Small sized nitinol baskets became possible that could be used to reliably access lower pole stones ureteroscopically, making it possible to grasp and relocate them to the upper pole for fragmentation with the holmium:YAG laser.

6.2. Variety of Stone Baskets

There are now a variety of stone baskets available for use, and the majority of manufacturers prefer nitinol as the primary element in design due to its responsiveness, kink resistance and negligible effect on the active deflection of flexible ureteroscopes [33]. The basket designs range from paired wires to spherical designs to complex woven wire net configurations, and generally, their use is based on the surgeon's preference. Table 5 shows the most commonly used nitinol baskets.

For routine use, we now prefer the Escape® (Boston Scientific) 1.9 Fr basket for the extraction of stone fragments in the ureter and renal pelvis. These baskets were made of two long wires which can open widely from 11 mm to 15 mm. For stones in a calyx, we use the N-Gage® (Cook) 1.7 Fr basket.

Table 5. The commonly available stone baskets

Manufacturer	Product name	Size (Fr)	Open diameters (mm)	length (cm)	Configuration
Cook	NCircle	1.5, 2.2, 3.0, 4.5	10, 20	115, 65	spherical
	NCircle Delta Wire	2.4	10, 20	115	spherical
	NCircle Helical	3.0, 4.5	10, 15	115, 65	helical
	NForce	2.2, 3.2	n/a	115	helical
	NGage	1.7, 2.2	8, 11	115	other
	NCompass	1.7, 2.4	10, 15	115	other
Boston Scientific	Zerotip	1.9, 2.4, 3.0	12, 16	90, 120	spherical
	Escape	1.9	11-15	90, 120	spherical
	Optiflex	1.3	6-11	90, 120	spherical
Coloplast-Porges	Dormia No-Tip	1.5, 2.2, 3.0	9, 11, 14	120, 90	spherical
	Dormia N. stone	2.5, 3, 4	12.5, 15	90	helical
Bard	Dimension	2.4, 3.0	10, 13, 16		spherical

It has a uniquely designed shape, which can easily grasp and release a stone in front of the scope. The 11 mm N-Gage basket is a preferred basket for the displacement of a large lower pole stone to the upper pole. The Dormia No-Tip® (Coloplast-Porges) 1.5 Fr is a small sized basket, which maintains good irrigation flow. It has a proper stiffness which makes it easy to handle.

Stone baskets are crucial to the endourologist's armamentarium. The instruments have evolved significantly as more advanced and miniaturized flexible ureteroscopes have been developed. With proper technique and a good knowledge of the stone baskets, it is possible to achieve complete stone-free status immediately after surgery.

7. Ureteral Stents

Ureteral stents are commonly used in urology to provide urinary drainage of the kidney or to splint a ureteral anastomosis. Ureteral stents are also used to decompress acute obstruction from a kidney stone until definitive therapy can be utilized to treat the stone.

Stents are also commonly left after the treatment for urolithiasis. The decision must be made at the end of ureteroscopy as to whether or not a ureteral stent should be placed. In the case of a perforation of the ureter or collecting system, ureteral stents should always be placed. Ureteral stents should also be placed in obviously infected cases, which may develop postoperative pyelonephritis. In addition, in the case in which adequate access cannot be achieved that require passive dilation of the ureter, ureteral stents are also indicated. Moreover, ureteral stents should also be placed in patients with a solitary kidney and severe hydronephrosis. In the case of bilateral ureteroscopy, we prefer to place ureteral stents bilaterally.

There have been many randomized clinical trials that have provided evidence that patients without ureteral stents have less postoperative pain and problems than those who receive a ureteral stent [34-36]. Patients without a ureteral stent tend to have fewer emergency room visits and to have less postoperative pain. These studies showed that patients who were randomized not to receive a stent after uncomplicated ureteroscopy did not have any more unexpected medical visits or requirements for stent insertion than patients who were stented postoperatively. However, there is also evidence to support the role for ureteral stenting following ureteroscopy. Borboroglu et al. reported that the risk of admission for flank pain post-ureteroscopy was 7.4% in the unstented versus a 0% readmission rate in the stented group [37]. However, in this same study, the unstented patients did have significantly less flank pain overall. Although leaving a stent is justified to prevent the development of ureteral strictures, a meta-analysis of randomized controlled trials by Nabi et al. indicated no difference in the stricture rate between stented and unstented patients [38]. Although many studies have shown fewer symptoms and less pain in the patients without a stent, a meta-analysis found a trend towards fewer urological complications in the patients who received a stent following ureteroscopy [39].

Therefore, the significance of postoperative stenting is controversial. We currently routinely place a stent for seven days after ureteroscopic surgery with either semirigid or flexible ureteroscopy. Postoperative stenting has some merits for surgeons. For example, even if a high grade fever occurs after the surgery, there need be no concerns about unintended ureteral damage, inducing extravasation of the urine or acute stricture of the ureter, which would require emergency drainage procedures. Additionally, we expect a passive dilation effect on the ureter and improved spontaneous passage of stone fragments. We also expect a preventive benefit for late stricture of the ureter in cases treated with stents.

7.1. Stent Biomaterials

Although there are a variety of different biomaterials used in stent design, the most popular biomaterial is a variation or combination involving polyurethane. Most are proprietary polymers based on this technology. Polyethylene stents, which were used originally, are no longer used today due to their stiffness and brittleness, which led to a tendency for them to fracture when left indwelling for a long periods of time. Newer blends of polyethylene and other polymers, such as polyurethane, have been developed to withstand the conditions of the urinary environment, and are more resistant to fracturing, encrusting and causing infections. Silicone is currently one of the most commonly used biocompatible materials today in terms of avoiding infection, encrustation and biofilm production. It is also very lubricious, which makes insertion easier and may potentially help with patient comfort; however, silicone's flexibility and elasticity are also the cause of the problems associated with silicone. Namely, negotiating silicone ureteral stents through narrow or tortuous ureters is very difficult. The findings based on the use of the brittle and firm polyethylene and soft silicone led to the use of polyurethane, which is a compromise between these two extremes. Polyurethane is the most common biomaterial used in ureteral stents today. Although it is the most commonly used, it is also fairly firm and is prone to causing significant discomfort in patients. Newer materials are constantly being developed, and include many proprietary polymers from various companies. The future of stent materials will likely include technologies to improve the patients' comfort while reducing encrustation, infection and maintaining the drainage characteristics. Newer coatings that will resist infection and encrustation will allow for longer indwelling of ureteral stents without sequelae.

7.2. Stent-Associated Discomfort

The most common complication of an indwelling ureteral stent is pain experienced by the patient. Over 80% of patients with a ureteral stent experience pain and discomfort [40]. Much speculation has gone into the cause of discomfort, and the exact causes are currently unknown, but one theory is uroepithelial irritation during stent movement within the ureter as the patient goes about their day-to-day activities. A previous study showed that the ureteral stent moves within the ureter, kidney and bladder when the patient moves, and may thus cause discomfort [41]. This movement is likely attributable to the fact that ureteral JJ-stents are not anchored in place: the pigtail curls in the bladder and kidney are designed to prevent migration of the stent, but still allow the stent to slide and move.

Even though there is no clear data to support the use of one type of stent over another, there is good data that longer stents that protrude into the bladder produce more symptoms. Choosing the correct length of stent will significantly improve the patient's stent-related symptoms. Stents that cross the midline of the bladder result in significantly more dysuria, urgency and irritative voiding symptoms than those that do not cross the midline. Fluoroscopic studies of stented patients showed that, with motion, the stent tends to bow in the mid and proximal ureter, and the excess length slides in and out of the bladder at the ureterovesical junction, with relatively little motion seen in the kidney [41].

Conclusion

It is important to understand the history of the developments of ureteroscopes and associated instruments. The problems associated with the current instruments should be taken into consideration, and efforts to solve these problems and develop next-generation instruments should be made.

References

[1] Young HH, Mckay RW. Congenital valvular obstruction of the prostatic urethra. *Surg. Gynecol. Obstet.* 1929; 48: 509-12.
[2] Marshal VV. Fiberoptics in urology. *J. Urol.* 1964; 91: 110-3.
[3] Goodman T. Ureteroscopy with pediatric cystoscope in adults. *Urology.* 1977; 9: 394.
[4] Lyon ES, Kyker JS, Schoenberg HW. Transurethral ureteroscopy in women: A ready addition to the urological armamentarium. *J. Urol.* 1978; 119: 35-6.
[5] Perez-Castro EE, Martinez-Piniero JA. Transurethral ureteroscopy- a current urological procedure. *Arch. Esp. Urol.* 1980; 33: 445-60.
[6] Takagi T, Go T, Takayasu N, Aso Y. Small-caliber fiberscope for visualization of the urinary tract, biliary tract, and spinal canal. *Surgery* 1968; 64: 1033-8.
[7] Seldinger SI. Catheter replacement of the needle in percutaneous arteriography; a new technique. *Acta Radiol.* 1953; 39: 368-76.
[8] Fritzsche P, Moorhead JD, Axford PD, et al. Urologic applications of angiographic guide wire and catheter techniques. *J. Urol.* 1981; 125: 774-80.
[9] Takayasu H, Aso Y. Recent development for pyeloureteroscopy: guide tube method for its introduction into the ureter. *J. Urol.* 1971; 112: 176-8.
[10] Kourambas J, Byrne RR, Preminger GM. Does a ureteral access sheath facilitate ureteroscopy? *J. Urol.* 2001; 165: 789-93.
[11] Delvecchio FC, Auge BK, Brizuela RM, et al. Assessment of stricture formation with the ureteral access sheath. *Urology.* 2003; 61: 518-22.
[12] Bilgasem S, Pace KT, Dyer S, et al. Removal of asymptomatic ipsilateral renal stones following rigid ureteroscopy for ureteral stones. *J. Endourol.* 2003; 17: 397-400.

[13] Chow GK, Patterson DE, Blute ML, et al. Ureteroscopy: effect of technology and technique on clinical practice. *J. Urol.* 2003; 170: 99-102.
[14] Harmon WJ, Sershon PD, Blute ML, et al. Ureteroscopy: current practice and long-term complications. *J. Urol.* 1997; 157: 28-32.
[15] Schuster TG, Hollenbeck BK, Faerber GJ, et al. Ureteroscopic treatment of lower pole calculi: comparison of lithotripsy in situ and after displacement. *J. Urol.* 2002; 168: 43-5.
[16] Sofer M, Watterson JD, Wollin TA, et al. Holmium: YAG laser lithotripsy for upper urinary tract calculi in 598 patients. *J. Urol.* 2002; 167: 31-4.
[17] L'esperance JO, Ekeruo WO, Scales Jr CD, et al. Effect of ureteral access sheath on stone-free rates in patients undergoing ureteroscopic management of renal calculi. *Urology.* 2005; 66: 252-5.
[18] Schwalb DM, Eshghi M, Davidian M, et al. Morphological and physiological changes in the urinary tract associated with ureteral dilation and ureteropyeloscopy: an experimental study. *J. Urol.* 1993; 149: 1576-85.
[19] Landman J, Venkatesh R, Ragab M, et al. Comparison of intrarenal pressure and irrigation flow during percutaneous nephroscopy with an indwelling ureteral catheter, ureteral occlusion balloon, and ureteral access sheath. *Urology.* 2002; 60: 584-7.
[20] Rehman J, Monga M, Landman J, et al. Characterization of intrapelvic pressure during ureteropyeloscopy with ureteral access sheaths. *Urology.* 2003; 61: 713-8.
[21] Lullas CD, Auge BK, Raj GV, et al. Laser Doppler flowmetric determination of ureteral blood flow after ureteral access sheath placement. *J. Endourol.* 2002; 16: 583-90.
[22] Cybulski P, Honey RJ, Pace K, et al. Fluid absorption during ureteroscopy. *J. Endourol.* 2004; 18: 739-42.
[23] Kukreja RA, Desai MR, Sabnis RB, et al. Fluid absorption during percutaneous nephrolithotomy: does it matter? *J. Endourol.* 2002; 16: 221-4.
[24] Holst U, Dissing T, Rawashdeh YF, et al. Norepinephrine inhibits the pelvic pressure increase in response to flow perfusion. *J. Urol.* 2003; 170: 268-71.
[25] Holst U, Rawashdeh YF, Andreasen F, et al. Endoluminal pelvic perfusion with norepinephrine causes only minor systemic effects and

diminishes the increase in pelvic pressure caused by perfusion. *Scand. J. Urol. Nephrol.* 2005; 39: 443-8.

[26] Jung HU, Jakobsen JS, Mortensen J, et al. Irrigation with isoproterenol diminishes increases in pelvic pressure without side-effects during ureterorenoscopy: a randomized controlled study in a porcine model. *Scand. J. Urol. Nephrol.* 2008; 42: 7-11.

[27] Danuser H, Weiss R, Abel D, et al. Systemic and topical drug administration in the pig ureter: effect of phosphodiesterase inhibitors alpha1, beta and beta2-adrenergic receptor agonists and antagonists on the frequency and amplitude of ureteral contractions. *J. Urol.* 2001; 166: 714-20.

[28] Jakobsen JS, Holst U, Jakobsen P, et al. Local and systemic effects of endoluminal pelvic perfusion of isoproterenol: a dose response investigation in pigs. *J. Urol.* 2007; 177: 1934-8.

[29] Selmy GI, Hassouna MM, Khalaf IM, et al. Effects of verapamil, prostaglandin F2 alpha, phenylephrine, and noradrenaline on upper urinary tract dynamics. *Urology.* 1994; 43: 31-5.

[30] Denstedt JD, Razvi HA, Sales JL, et al. Preliminary experience with holmium:YAG laser lithotripsy. *J. Endourol.* 1995; 9: 255-8.

[31] Sea J, Jonat LM, Chew BH, et al. Optimal power settings for holmium:YAG lithotripsy. *J. Urol.* 2012; 187: 914-9.

[32] Honey RJD'A. Assessment of a new tipless nitinol stone basket and comparison with an existing flat wire basket. *J. Endourol.* 1998; 12: 529-31.

[33] Leone NT, Garcia-Roig M, Bagley DH. Changing trends in the use of ureteroscopic instruments from 1996 to 2008. *J. Endourol.* 2010; 24: 361-5.

[34] Chen YT, Chen J, Wong WY, et al. Is ureteral stenting necessary after uncomplicated ureteroscopic lithotripsy? A prospective, randomized controlled trial. *J. Urol.* 2002; 167: 1977-80.

[35] Hussein A, Rifaat E, Zaki A, et al. Stenting versus non-stenting after non-complicated ureteroscopic manipulation of stones in biharzial ureters. *Int. J. Urol.* 2006; 13: 886-90.

[36] Isen K, Bogatekin S, Em S, et al. Is routine ureteral stenting necessary after uncomplicated ureteroscopic lithotripsy for lower ureteral stones larger than 1 cm? *Urol. Res.* 2008; 36: 115-9.

[37] Borboroglu PG, Amling CL, Schenkman NS, et al. Ureteral stenting after ureteroscopy for distal ureteral calculi: a multi-institutional

prospective randomized controlled study assessing pain, outcomes and complications. *J. Urol.* 2001; 166: 1651-7.

[38] Nabi G, Cook J, N'Dow J, et al. Outcomes of stenting after uncomplicated ureteroscopy: systematic review and meta-analysis. *BMJ.* 2007; 334: 572.

[39] Makarov DV, Trock BJ, Allaf ME, et al. The effect of ureteral stent placement on post-ureteroscopy complications: a meta-analysis. *Urology* 2008; 71: 796-800.

[40] Joshi HB, Stainthorpe A, MacDonagh RP, et al. Indwelling ureteral stents: evaluation of symptoms, quality of life and utility. *J. Urol.* 2003; 169: 1065-9.

[41] Chew BH, Knudsen BE, Nott L, et al. Pilot study of ureteral movement in stented patients: first step in understanding dynamic ureteral anatomy to improve stent comfort. *J. Endourol.* 2007; 21: 1069-75.

PART III. TECHNIQUES

Chapter 3

Preoperative Preparation: Antibiotics, Prestenting, and Percutaneous Nephrostomy

Takashi Kawahara[*], M.D.[1,2,3], Hiroki Ito, M.D.[1,2],*
Hiroji Uemura, M.D., Ph.D.[2],
Yoshinobu Kubota, M.D., Ph.D.[2]
Junichi Matsuzaki, M.D., Ph.D.[1]

[1]Department of Urology, Ohguchi Higashi General Hospital, Japan
[2]Department of Urology, Yokohama City University
Graduate School of Medicine, Japan
[3]Departments of Pathology and Urology,
Johns Hopkins University School of Medicine, Baltimore, Maryland, US

Abstaract

Large renal stones can be treated ureteroscopically, although more than one procedure is often required. The reason for this is that a longer operative time is associated with postoperative urinary tract infection (UTI). The use of stenting prior to URS was recently reported, with good

---

[*] Corresponding author: Takashi Kawahara, M.D. takashi_tk2001@yahoo.co.jp.

efficacy in improving the stone-free rate. In addition, percutaneous nephrostomy is effective for reducing the incidence of complications, as the procedure contributes to decreasing the intrarenal pressure. Furthermore, the administration of preoperative antibiotics reduces the rate postoperative UTI.

Our findings showed that preoperative stenting is effective for dilating the ureter and facilitating the insertion of a ureteral access sheath in patients undergoing ureteroscopic lithotripsy for large renal stones.

Introduction

When performing URS, preoperative preparation is effective in improving the operative efficacy and preventing URS-related complications. In this section, we describe the protocol for preoperative preparation, including the use of preoperative antibiotics, preoperative stenting and percutaneous nephrostomy.

1. Preoperative Antibiotics

Ureteroscopic lithotripsy is a widely used procedure to treat patients with ureteral stones. Most objective patients have obstruction in the upper urinary tract, such as stones, tumors or stricture in the ureter [1, 2]. Matsumoto et al. reported that postoperative UTI easily occurs, sometimes progressing to febrile UTI, in cases involving obstruction and/or invasive procedures. Therefore, the administration of preoperative antibiotics during these procedures is necessary. The incidence of perioperative infection ranges from 3.9% to 10%, depending on the operative invasiveness, in other words the difficulty of the procedure [3, 4, 5, 6. Preoperative prophylactic antibiotic therapy plays an important role in reducing postoperative surgical site infection. However, only a few randomized controlled trials have compared the efficacy of different regimens of prophylactic antibiotics in preventing surgical site infection after ureteroscopic lithotripsy [2, 7, 8, 9].

Hsieh et al. conducted a randomized controlled study to assess the impact of preoperative antibiotics in among patients undergoing ureteroscopic lithotripsy divided into four groups, including those receiving oral levofloxacin (500 mg), intravenous cefazolin (1 g), ceftriaxone (1 g) or no preoperative antibiotics. The authors reported that, although there were no significant differences in the rate of postoperative fever between the different antibiotic groups, levofloxacin and ceftriaxone were associated with a lower incidence of postoperative pyuria [2].

2. Prestenting

2.1. What Is Prestenting?

Previous reports have found that prestenting improves the rate of successful ureteroscopic lithotripsy [10-12]. Ureteral stenting helps to dilate the ureter, which results in easy access to the renal collecting system. In most of these reports, preoperative stenting was performed for passive reasons, such as to protect the renal function and avoid pain or treat urosepsis. Chu et al. showed that prestenting is associated with a decreased operative time and rate of reoperation in patients with a large stone burden of > 1 cm [11]. In previous reports regarding the effectiveness of prestenting in adult patients, the reasons for stenting were almost all passive, including treatment for urosepsis and to avoid pain and/or protect the renal function from hydronephrosis [10-12].

2.2. Intentional Prestenting

On the other hand, some reports sought to perform preoperative stenting in order to improve the effectiveness of ureteroscopy [13-15]. The stone burden is a reliable predictor of whether the stone is free during ureteroscopic lithotripsy. In addition, a stone burden of 23.0 mm has been proposed as a cut-off point for achieving a stone-free status [16]. Therefore, patients with large urinary stones measuring approximately 20.0 mm are potential candidates for acquiring a stone-free status using a single ureteroscopic procedure.

2.3. Which Type of Stent?

Types of Ureteral Stents

Ureteral stents contain various materials and are available in different sizes, coatings and shapes to avoid unpleasant urinary symptoms and discomfort [17-19]. It is necessary to minimize the amount material in the bladder in order to decrease stent-related symptoms [17]. Therefore, the Tail Stent® (Boston Scientific, USA) was developed with a 7-Fr proximal pigtail and 7-Fr shaft that tapers to a lumenless straight 3-Fr tail at the distal end [20]. Dunn et al. showed that 7-Fr tail loop stents produce significantly less irritating symptoms than standard 7-Fr double-pigtail stents. Lingeman et al. assessed stent-related symptoms associated with various types of ureteral stents using a self-administered questionnaire. Loop-type ureteral stents were found to exhibit lower stent-related symptom scores than standard double stents, although not significantly [21]. We investigated the effectiveness of changing to a loop-type ureteral stent among a total of 25 patients with a median age of 56.5 years (52.9 ± 12.2) who underwent ureteral stent exchange [22]. Almost all stent-related symptoms not associated with nocturia demonstrated significantly lower scores in the loop-type ureteral stent group than in the double-pigtail stent group. With respect to the ureteral stent position, the symptom score was differentiated by the stent placed in the distal end. When the shaft of the stent was placed across the midline, the symptom score was higher than that observed when the shaft was placed fully within the ureter. Therefore, it is necessary to select the appropriate length of ureteral stent. In addition, changing to a loop-type ureteral stent significantly decreases the rate of ureteral stent-related symptoms.

Length of Ureteral Stent

Changing to a loop-type ureteral stent significantly decreases the incidence of ureteral stent-related symptoms [22]. However, inserting an inappropriate length of ureteral stent is meaningless. Choosing the optimal length of ureteral stent is important for decreasing the incidence of stent migration and other complications [23-26] [27], [28] [28]. We therefore investigated the correlation between the ureteral length and ureteral stent length among 226 patients treated with loop-type ureteral stents using direct ureteral length measurements. Nine stents (3.9%) were found to have migrated, 171 stents (75.7%) were located in the appropriate position and 46 stents (19.5%) were too long. We placed ureteral stents that were the same length as the ureter; however, 10 of 91 stents (11.0%) were found to be longer than the ureter when the proximal ureteral stent was placed in the renal pelvis. Direct measurement with a ureteral catheter is thought to be the optimal method for selecting the appropriate length of ureteral stent. The appropriate length of ureteral stent is the same as or -1 cm less than the measured ureteral length. The use of ureteral stents more than 2 cm smaller than the measured ureteral length is associated with an increased incidence of migration. The insertion of a ureteral stent 1 cm shorter than the measured ureteral length is ideal, with a 2.6% risk of migration and 8.6% risk of being too long.

Choosing a ureteral stent via direct measurement of the ureteral length is ideal, although both the patient and operator are exposed to additional radiation and an extra procedure is required. Therefore, it is necessary to estimate the ureteral length. The correlation with the patient's height is generally used to estimate the ureteral length. However, the reliability of this method for estimating the ureteral length has not yet been confirmed [29]. A variety of tools for determining the actual ureteral length have been reported, including: (1) the patient's body height, (2) variables of the body habitus, (3) direct measurement of the ureter using a ureteral catheter, (4) direct measurement using a guidewire, (5) ureteral tracing using intravenous urography (IVU), (6) measurement of the distance from the ureteropelvic junction (UPJ) to the ureterovesical junction (UVJ) on IVU and (7) measurement of the distance from the mid kidney to UVJ on IVU [30-33]. We previously analyzed patients who underwent both preoperative IVU and CT. In that study, the ureteral length was measured using a ruled 5-Fr ureteral catheter (TigerTail®, BARD, USA) in 151 Japanese patients (94 males, 57 females, 169 ureters), and the correlations between the following factors and the actual ureteral length were assessed: and (1) body height (BH), (2) body surface area (BSA), (3) ureteral tracing (UT) on IVU, (4) linear distance (Linear Distance 1: LD1) from the UPJ to the UVJ on IVU, (5) linear distance (Linear Distance 2: LD2) from the mid-kidney to the UVJ on IVU and (6) the distance from the level of the renal vein to the UVJ on non-contrast axial computed tomography (CT) (axial CT distance: ACTD). The correlation coefficients for BH, BSA, UT, LD1, LD2 and ACTD were 0.3258, 0.3255, 0.4917, 0.5413, 0.5265 and 0.6124, respectively.

The ACTD values correlated best with the actual ureteral length, as predicted by the Spearman correlation. The AUL was calculated for each variable, respectively: BH-AUL (cm): 0.0687 x BH (cm) + 12.05. BSA-AUL (cm): 3.3167 x BSA (m^2) + 17.69. UT-AUL (cm): 0.3739 x UT (cm) + 13.94. LD1-AUL (cm): 0.398 x LD1 (cm) + 13.71. LD2-AUL (cm): 0.4134 x LD2 (cm) + 12.56. ACTD-AUL (cm): 0.044 x ACTD (mm) + 13.25. The ACTD was therefore found to predict the actual ureteral length better than BH, BSA or IVU and to be a reliable predictor of ureteral length. Therefore, although directly measuring the ureteral length is ideal, ACTD is a potential new option for estimating the ureteral length and thus choosing the appropriate length of ureteral stent.

2.4. When to Perform Prestenting?

In previous studies, intentional prestenting was performed in children one or two weeks prior to URS [14, 15]. In our institute, preoperative prestenting is performed 7-20 days before URS. Stent placement can result in unpleasant side effects, such as urinary frequency, urgency, incontinence, hematuria and bladder and flank pain, which have a negative impact on the patient's quality of life [34]. In addition, although the rate of ureteral stent encrustation increases in association with the indwelling time, 42.8% of irremovable ureteral stents are detected within four months [35, 36]. Our previous report showed no differences in the stone-free rate (< 4 mm) in relation to the stent indwelling time [13]. Therefore, 7-10 days is adequate for dilating and straightening the ureter prior to ureteroscopic lithotripsy.

2.5. Criteria for Prestenting

The criteria for prestenting are important. Not all patients require prestenting before URS. Our previous reports showed that prestenting increases the stone-free rate from 27.8% to 44.0% (+16.2%) as well as the rate of completion during the initial operation from 55.6% to 72.0% (+16.4%). In other words, 83.8% of patients are not affected by prestenting in terms of the stone-free status and 8.36% of patients are not affected in terms of the completion of the initial operation. We therefore believe that intentional prestenting is only effective in patients with large renal stones, measuring approximately 20 mm.

3. Percutaneous Nephrostomy

Percutaneous nephrostomy is a useful tool for performing URS, as nephrostomy decreases the intrarenal pressure. Usually, the irrigation flow is restricted so as not to induce a postoperative UTI; thus, it is sometimes difficult to obtain a higher degree of visualization.

On the other hand, PCNL is easily performed in patients treated with nephrostomy. Therefore, the presence of renal stones measuring more than 2 cm may not be a good criterion for performing ureteroscopy with nephrostomy.

Since 1955, percutaneous nephrostomy has been a standard procedure for achieving urinary diversion in the management of postrenal obstruction or as a prelude to endourological procedures [37-41]. The efficacy of percutaneous nephrostomy in decompressing areas of urinary obstruction associated with infection caused by ureteral stones has been firmly established. Furthermore, percutaneous nephrostomy shows a high rate of success and low incidence of complications [37, 42].

PCNL is an established procedure that provides temporary or permanent drainage for an obstructed urinary system. PCNL is primarily performed to treat urinary stones, urinary tract infection, acute renal failure and severe flank pain due to urinary tract obstruction [37, 43-45]. Therefore, patients may undergo flexible URS in the presence of percutaneous nephrostomy [37].

Kwon et al. reported that the use of flexible ureteroscopy in the presence of PCN produces superior outcomes in terms of the success rate, without increasing the operative time or complication rate [37].

Conclusion

When performing URS, the administration of preoperative antibiotics is useful for preventing postoperative UTIs. Performing URS is easy in patients with ureteral stents. In some cases, the use of intentional prestenting and/or percutaneous nephrostomy is helpful for treating large renal stones.

References

[1] Matsumoto, T., et al., Japanese guidelines for prevention of perioperative infections in urological field. *Int. J. Urol.* 2007; 14: 890-909.

[2] Hsieh, C.H., et al., Is Prophylactic Antibiotics Necessary in Patients with Pre-operative Sterile Urine Undergoing Ureteroscopic Lithotripsy? *BJU Int*, 2013.

[3] Grabe, M., Perioperative antibiotic prophylaxis in urology. *Curr. Opin. Urol.* 2001; 11: 81-5.

[4] Puppo, P., et al., Primary endoscopic treatment of ureteric calculi. A review of 378 cases. *Eur. Urol.* 1999; 36: 48-52.

[5] Larsen, E.H., T.C. Gasser, and P.O. Madsen, Antimicrobial prophylaxis in urologic surgery. *Urol. Clin. North. Am.* 1986; 13: 591-604.
[6] Rao, P.N., et al., Prediction of septicemia following endourological manipulation for stones in the upper urinary tract. *J. Urol.* 1991;.146: 955-60.
[7] Fourcade, R.O., Antibiotic prophylaxis with cefotaxime in endoscopic extraction of upper urinary tract stones: a randomized study. The Cefotaxime Cooperative Group. *J. Antimicrob. Chemother.* 1990; 26 Suppl A: 77-83.
[8] Christiano, A.P., et al., Double-blind randomized comparison of single-dose ciprofloxacin versus intravenous cefazolin in patients undergoing outpatient endourologic surgery. *Urology.* 2000; 55: 182-5.
[9] Knopf, H.J., H.J. Graff, and H. Schulze, Perioperative antibiotic prophylaxis in ureteroscopic stone removal. *Eur. Urol.* 2003; 44: 115-8.
[10] Shields, J.M., et al., Impact of preoperative ureteral stenting on outcome of ureteroscopic treatment for urinary lithiasis. *J. Urol.* 2009; 182: 2768-74.
[11] Chu, L., K.M. Sternberg, and T.D. Averch, Preoperative stenting decreases operative time and reoperative rates of ureteroscopy. *J. Endourol.* 2011; 25: 751-4.
[12] Rubenstein, R.A., et al., Prestenting improves ureteroscopic stone-free rates. *J. Endourol.* 2007; 21: 1277-80.
[13] Kawahara, T., et al., Preoperative stenting for ureteroscopic lithotripsy for a large renal stone. *Int. J. Urol.* 2012; 19: 881-5.
[14] Hubert, K.C. and J.S. Palmer, Passive dilation by ureteral stenting before ureteroscopy: eliminating the need for active dilation. *J. Urol.* 2005; 174: 1079-80.
[15] Corcoran, A.T., et al., When is prior ureteral stent placement necessary to access the upper urinary tract in prepubertal children? *J. Urol.* 2008; 180(4 Suppl): 1861-3.
[16] Ito, H., et al., The most reliable preoperative assessment of renal stone burden as a predictor of stone-free status after flexible ureteroscopy with holmium laser lithotripsy: a single-center experience. *Urology.* 2012; 80: 524-8.
[17] Lingeman, J.E., et al., Assessing the impact of ureteral stent design on patient comfort. *J. Urol.* 2009. 181: 2581-7.
[18] Joshi, H.B., et al., A prospective randomized single-blind comparison of ureteral stents composed of firm and soft polymer. *J. Urol.* 2005; 174: 2303-6.

[19] Dellis, A., et al., Relief of stent related symptoms: review of engineering and pharmacological solutions. *J. Urol.* 2010; 184: 1267-72.
[20] Dunn, M.D., et al., Clinical effectiveness of new stent design: randomized single-blind comparison of tail and double-pigtail stents. *J. Endourol.* 2000; 14: 195-202.
[21] Lingeman, J.E., et al., Assessing the impact of ureteral stent design on patient comfort. *J. Urol.* 2009; 181: 2581-7.
[22] Kawahara, T., et al., Changing to a loop-type ureteral stent decreases patients' stent-related symptoms. *Urol. Res.* 2012; 40: 763-7.
[23] Wills, M.I., et al., Which ureteric stent length? *Br. J. Urol.* 1991; 68: 440.
[24] Pocock, R.D., et al., Double J stents. A review of 100 patients. *Br. J. Urol.* 1986; 58: 629-33.
[25] Chin, J.L. and J.D. Denstedt, Retrieval of proximally migrated ureteral stents. *J. Urol.* 1992; 148: 1205-6.
[26] Slaton, J.W. and K.A. Kropp, Proximal ureteral stent migration: an avoidable complication? *J. Urol.* 1996; 155: 58-61.
[27] Kawahara, T., et al., Choosing an appropriate length of loop type ureteral stent using direct ureteral length measurement. *Urol. Int.* 2012; 88: 48-53.
[28] Kawahara, T., et al., Which is the best method to estimate the actual ureteral length in patients undergoing ureteral stent placement? *Int. J. Urol.* 2012; 19: 634-8.
[29] Shah, J. and R.P. Kulkarni, Height does not predict ureteric length. *Clin. Radiol.* 2005; 60: 812-4.
[30] Pilcher, J.M. and U. Patel, Choosing the correct length of ureteric stent: a formula based on the patient's height compared with direct ureteric measurement. *Clin. Radiol.* 2002; 57: 59-62.
[31] Paick, S.H., et al., Direct ureteric length measurement from intravenous pyelography: does height represent ureteric length? *Urologic. Res.* 2005; 33: 199-202.
[32] Hruby, G.W., et al., Correlation of ureteric length with anthropometric variables of surface body habitus. *BJU Int.* 2007; 99: 1119-22.
[33] Ho, C.H., et al., Choosing the ideal length of a double-pigtail ureteral stent according to body height: study based on a Chinese population. *Urol. Int.* 2009; 83: 70-4.
[34] Ho, C.H., et al., Choosing the ideal length of a double-pigtail ureteral stent according to body height: study based on a Chinese population. *Urol. Int.* 2009; 83: 70-4.

[35] Bultitude, M.F., et al., Management of encrusted ureteral stents impacted in upper tract. *Urology.* 2003; 62: 622-6.
[36] el-Faqih, S.R., et al., Polyurethane internal ureteral stents in treatment of stone patients: morbidity related to indwelling times. *J. Urol.* 1991, 146: 1487-91.
[37] Kwon, S.Y., et al., Efficacy of percutaneous nephrostomy during flexible ureteroscopy for renal stone management. *Korean. J.* Urol. 2013; 54: 689-92.
[38] Goodwin, W.E., W.C. Casey, and W. Woolf, Percutaneous trocar (needle) nephrostomy in hydronephrosis. *J. Am. Med. Assoc.* 1955; 157: 891-4.
[39] Montvilas, P., J. Solvig, and T.E. Johansen, Single-centre review of radiologically guided percutaneous nephrostomy using "mixed" technique: success and complication rates. *Eur. J. Radiol.* 2011; 80: 553-8.
[40] Lee, W.J., et al., Emergency percutaneous nephrostomy: results and complications. *J. Vasc. Interv. Radiol.* 1994; 5: 135-9.
[41] Bell, D.A., et al., Percutaneous nephrostomy for nonoperative management of fungal urinary tract infections. *J. Vasc. Interv. Radiol.* 1993; 4: 311-5.
[42] Mokhmalji, H., et al., Percutaneous nephrostomy versus ureteral stents for diversion of hydronephrosis caused by stones: a prospective, randomized clinical trial. *J. Urol.* 2001; 165: 1088-92.
[43] Dyer, R.B., et al., Percutaneous nephrostomy with extensions of the technique: step by step. *Radiographics.* 2002; 22: 503-25.
[44] Hausegger, K.A. and H.R. Portugaller, Percutaneous nephrostomy and antegrade ureteral stenting: technique-indications-complications. *Eur. Radiol.* 2006; 16: 2016-30.
[45] Avritscher, R., et al., Fistulas of the lower urinary tract: percutaneous approaches for the management of a difficult clinical entity. *Radiographics.* 2004; 24 Suppl 1: S217-36.

Chapter 4

Semirigid and Flexible Ureteroscopy: Ohtsuka Method

Ryoji Takazawa*, M.D., Ph.D., Sachi Kitayama, M.D. and Toshihiko Tsujii, M.D., Ph.D.*
Department of Urology, Tokyo Metropolitan Ohtsuka Hospital,
Tokyo, Japan

Abstract

Ureteroscopic lithotripsy is composed of several steps. First, the patient is positioned in an appropriate surgical position, and the instruments are set in the correct positions. After standard cystoscopy, a guidewire is inserted into the ureteral orifice and is advanced over the stones very carefully. A semirigid ureteroscope is then inserted over the working guidewire. In the case of flexible ureteroscopy, a ureteral access sheath is placed. Once the ureteroscope is advanced into the ureter, the stone can be visualized and fragmented by using a holmium:YAG laser. After the fragmentation, the stone pieces are removed systematically. After the removal of the stone fragments, a ureteral stent can be placed. In this chapter, we describe our routine techniques used for ureteroscopic lithotripsy.

---

[*] Corresponding author: Ryoji Takazawa, M.D., Ph.D. ryoji_takazawa@tmhp.jp.

Introduction

Ureteroscopic lithotripsy is composed of several steps. First, the patient is positioned in an appropriate surgical position, and the instruments are set in the correct positions. After standard cystoscopy, a guidewire is inserted into the ureteral orifice and is advanced very carefully over the stone(s). A semirigid ureteroscope is inserted over the working guidewire. In the case of flexible ureteroscopy, a ureteral access sheath is placed. Once the ureteroscope is advanced into the ureter, the stone can be visualized and fragmented by using a holmium: YAG laser. After completing the fragmentation, the stone pieces are removed systematically. After the removal of stone fragments, a ureteral stent can be placed. To achieve the successful treatments, surgeons have developed several common techniques. Moreover, based on their own experiments, surgeons exercise their ingenuity to achieve more successful outcomes. In this chapter, we describe our routine techniques used for ureteroscopic lithotripsy.

1. Patient Position and Room Settings

The patient is positioned in the dorsal lithotomy position where the legs are lowered and slightly extended [Figure 1a]. The patient should not be able to move during the insertion of a ureteroscope, because sudden patient movement could result in perforation or other complications. Therefore, a good degree of muscle relaxation with general anesthesia or an adequate level of spinal anesthesia is preferred.

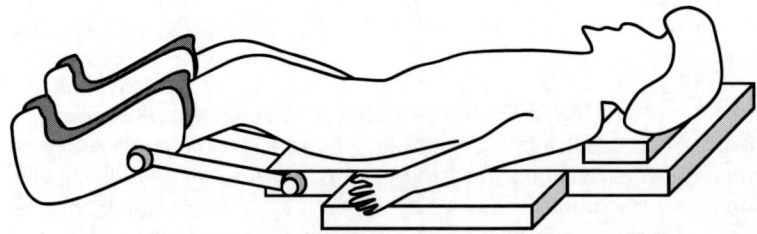

Figure 1a.

The C-arm is set up for intraoperative fluoroscopy. The light source, holmium laser and video and C-arm monitors are positioned on one side of the patient, and the C-arm is positioned on the contralateral side. If the patient's upper extremity interferes with the fluoroscopic equipment, the ipsilateral arm should be tucked away. Concurrent percutaneous nephrolithotomy (PCNL) is an example of an exception to the standard lithotomy position for ureteroscopy. We prefer to use the Galdakao-modified supine Valdivia position [Figure 1b], which facilitates both transurethral and percutaneous approaches, in cases where a combined procedure will be performed [1, 2]. This supine position has less anesthetic risks and comparable risks of splanchnic injury to the conventional prone position. The access field is more limited and the tract length is slightly longer, which may be a disadvantage for the maneuverability of the surgeon.

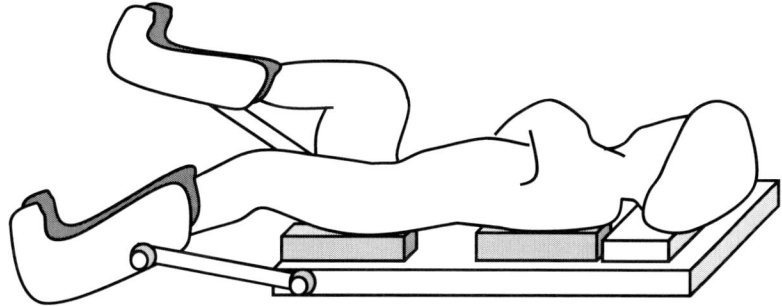

Figure 1b.

As a result, some experts prefer to use the prone split-leg position. This prone position provides a larger manipulation space and shorter tract length for percutaneous renal access, although the prone position may induce more anesthetic risk than the supine position [3, 4].

2. Semirigid Ureteroscopy

After the patient is prepared in the dorsal lithotomy position, standard cystoscopy is performed. At that time, the position and shape of the ureteral orifice should be checked. If no preexisting ureteral stent is in place, the ureteral orifice is cannulated with a 0.035-inch PTFE-coated stiff-shaft guidewire through a 5 or 6 Fr open-ended ureteral catheter. The guidewire should be advanced over the stone(s) very carefully. If difficulty is encountered during the insertion of a stiff-shaft guidewire due to either obstruction or tortuosity within the ureter, an angled-tip hydrophilic guidewire will often help to navigate the problematic segment. If necessary, retrograde pyeloureterography can be performed using radiographic contrast diluted 50:50 with normal saline. This may open the niche of the impacted stone. Then, if possible, we also insert an open-ended ureteral catheter over the stone(s) in order to decompress the intrarenal pressure. If a preexisting ureteral stent is present, the stent is brought out to the urethral meatus using graspers through the cystoscope, and then the urethra is cannulated with a 0.035-inch stiff-shaft guidewire in the same way.

We usually use a dual-channel semirigid ureteroscope. Over a working guidewire, the semirigid ureteroscope is inserted into the ureteral orifice. With a modern tapered semirigid ureteroscope, it is rare for a ureteral orifice to be overly narrow and restrict the insertion of the ureteroscope. But on occasion, we first use a 10 Fr dilating catheter. We do not place a safety guidewire when performed the procedure with a semirigid ureteroscope. We always handle the semirigid ureteroscope with a guidewire through a working channel, while utilizing a laser fiber or a basket catheter thorough another working channel [Figures 2a and 2b]. A single-action irrigation pump (SAPS-CF**R**, Boston Scientific) is utilized to provide pressure irrigation at the appropriate times.

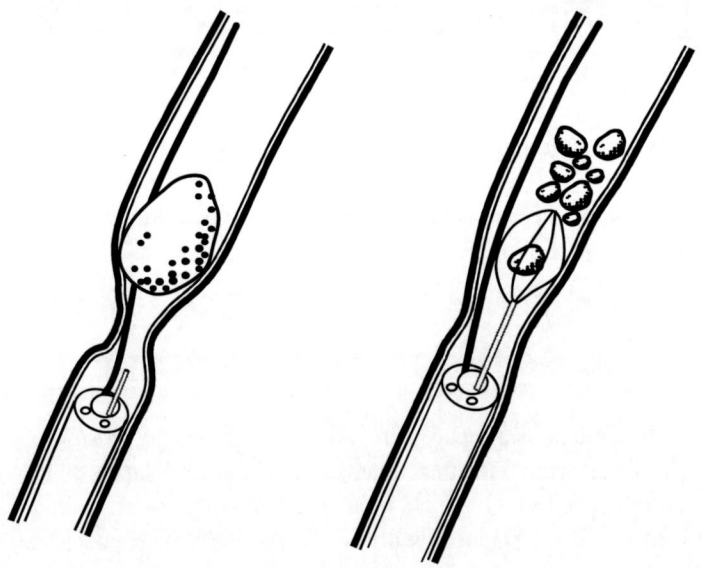

Figure 2a and b.

Once the ureteroscope is advanced into the ureter, the stone can be visualized and treated. The stone is fragmented by using a holmium:YAG laser. We generally use a 365 μm or 200 μm laser fiber. The power of the laser is set at 0.6-0.8 J and 6-8 Hz. We fragment the stone into pieces small enough to be removed with a stone basket. After catching the stone pieces with a stone basket, the ureteroscope is backed out of the ureter, bladder and urethra. The ureteroscope is reinserted over the working guidewire. This procedure is repeated until all of the stone pieces are cleared.

3. Flexible Ureteroscopy

We insert a ureteral access sheath (UAS) after the inspection with the semirigid ureteroscopy clears the ureter for unsuspected pathology. The UAS is particularly helpful, as it facilitates the repeated removal and reintroduction of the flexible ureteroscope into the upper urinary tract. It also protects a significant length of ureter from iatrogenic injury during this procedure. The use of access sheaths has been associated with improved stone-free rates, lower intraoperative intrarenal pressures and a shortened length of the operation. We can now utilize UAS of different sizes made by various manufactures. When selecting the size of the UAS, we usually try several sizes of dilators to determine whether they can be inserted without difficulty. We generally select a 12/14 Fr diameter UAS, although we sometimes use a 13/15 Fr or 14/16 Fr sheath in patient who have been pre-stented and have a large stone burden. If resistance is encountered during the insertion of the smaller ureteral access sheath (11/13 Fr or 10/12 Fr), we resort to a direct ureteroscopic insertion over a guidewire. For female patients, we select a 35 cm UAS. For males, we select either the 35 cm or 45 cm length, although the 45 cm UAS is sometimes difficult to insert. Once the UAS has been advanced into the ureter under fluoroscopic guidance, the inner dilator is removed along with the working guidewire, and the flexible ureteroscope is assembled. Despite some reports to the contrary, the use of a safety guidewire is advisable during flexible ureteroscopy, because complications such as ureteral perforation can occur even during uncomplicated procedures. Ureteral perforation necessitates prompt placement of a ureteral stent. In addition, a safety guidewire can keep the ureter straight and prevent ureteral perforation.

We basically utilize a fiberoptic flexible ureteroscope for lithotripsy. For the evaluation and treatment of upper tract urothelial carcinomas, the use of a digital Olympus flexible ureteroscope with narrow-band imaging capabilities has been demonstrated to improve cancer detection and the definition of margins for tumor ablation in comparison to white light imaging.

The Ho:YAG laser is the gold standard among intracorporeal lithotrites. The laser fibers should be advanced with the flexible endoscope undeflected so as to minimize the risk of trauma to the working channel. While the 365 μm fiber provides better durability and overall stone fragmentation, the 200 μm fiber better mitigates the reduction in deflection capability during flexible ureteroscopy. We prefer to use the 200 um fiber in flexible ureteroscopy. Typically, we will utilize a laser setting of 0.5-1.0 J and 6-10 Hz. We recommend increasing the frequency rather than the energy if the stone does not fragment sufficiently with an energy setting of 1.0 J, because lower energy settings lead to smaller stone fragments and less degradation of the laser fiber tip.

After fragmentation of the stone, the pieces are removed systematically. Care must be taken not to extract stones that are too large and to avoid injury to the ureter. There are a variety of stone removal devices available for use, and the majority of manufacturers prefer nitinol as the primary element in design due to its responsiveness, kink resistance and negligible effect on the active deflection of flexible scopes. The basket designs range from paired wires to spherical designs to complex woven wire net configurations, and generally, their use is based on the surgeon's preference. For routine use, we favor the tip-less circle type, which can easily capture and release the stone fragments. We select the small size (less than 1.9 Fr) basket because it permits better irrigation.

After the fragments are removed, the UAS is slowly withdrawn while the ureter is simultaneously inspected with the flexible ureteroscope. This is performed to ensure that no stones were missed in the ureter and that no other pathology of the ureter is present.

4. Postoperative Ureteral Stenting

After the removal of the UAS, we generally place a ureteral stent (4.7-6 Fr). The ureteral stent is left for about seven days in order to prevent postoperative ureteral stricture. Residual fragments are assessed with plain X-ray or CT scans. Then, the ureteral stent is removed when only small, if any, residual stones are confirmed. Otherwise, a second procedure is scheduled two to four weeks after the first procedure. After the removal of the ureteral stent, patients undergo renal ultrasound to ensure the stability of the upper urinary tracts.

5. Tips and Tricks

Access to the ureter can be challenging in a variety of situations. The first problem can occur when obtaining access to the ureteral orifice for intubation with the guidewire. Several problems and potential solutions will be presented below. Inflammation and distortion of the ureteral orifice from an impacted stone in the intramural tunnel can make the access difficult [Figure 3a]. In addition, a kinked ureter caused by an impacted stone at the ureterovesical junction can also make the access difficult [Figure 3b].

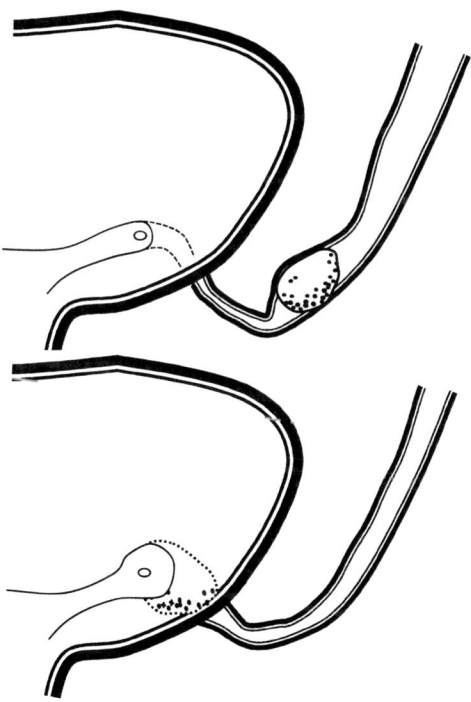

Figure 3a and b.

The use of an angled-tip hydrophilic-coated guidewire will often allow the wire to pass alongside the stone. This wire is quite slippery due to its hydrophilic nature, and thus, should not be utilized as a safety guidewire. A hydrophilic guidewire may become displaced more easily and compromise the ureteral access. If access is achieved with a hydrophilic guidewire, it should be exchanged, if possible, for a PTFE-coated stiff guidewire in order to prevent the loss of access.

A severely enlarged prostatic median lobe can make it difficult to reach the ureteral orifice with a rigid cystoscope. This can be overcome by using a flexible ureteroscope with an angled-tip hydrophilic-coated guidewire. In addition, if access to the ureter is achieved in such cases, a hydrophilic guidewire should be exchanged for a PTFE-coated stiff guidewire. A stiff guidewire will help hold the median lobe out of the way for passage of the semirigid ureteroscope. A severely trabeculated bladder can make identification of the ureteral orifice difficult, but can usually be helped by administering intravenous indigo carmine.

The next potential problem encountered is difficulty in passing the guidewire through the ureter into the kidney. This can be the result of an impacted ureteral stone [Figure 4a], ureteral stricture, ureteropelvic junction obstruction [Figure 4b] or a tortuous "kinked" ureter.

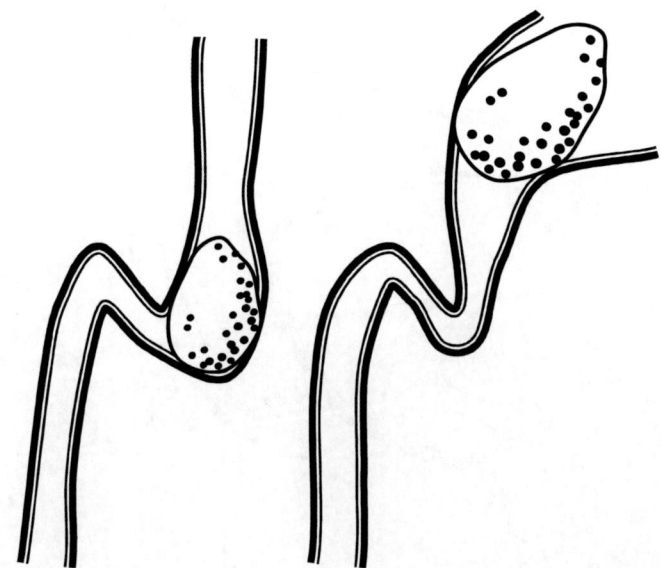

Figure 4a and b.

The use of an angled-tip hydrophilic-coated guidewire will often overcome this problem. Retrograde pyeloureterography may also open the niche of the impacted stone. If these are unsuccessful, direct ureteroscopic inspection, and if needed, fragmentation of the impacted stone, can be used to negotiate the guidewire around the point of obstruction [Figure 5]. Mid-ureteral stones are relatively uncommon. However, if the stone is impacted at mid-ureter, there may be difficulties with treatment because of the presence of severe edematous mucosa or ureteral stricture, which obstructs the spontaneous stone expulsion [Figure 6].

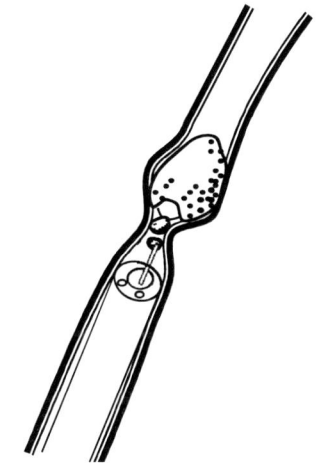

Figure 5.

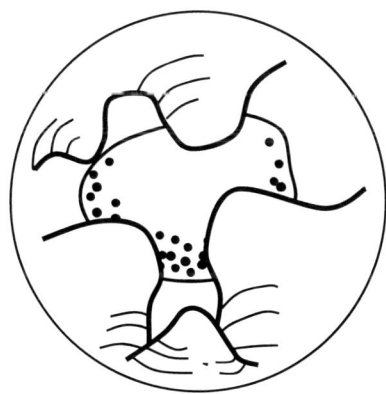

Figure 6.

Once the guidewire has been placed, the passage of the semirigid ureteroscope is usually straightforward, but can be hindered by several problems. It is important to keep the guidewire, over which the semirigid ureteroscope is passed, taut. Any slack in this guidewire will prevent the successful passage of the ureteroscope. Rotating the semirigid ureteroscope can help present a more streamlined face of the ureteroscope to the ureteral orifice [Figure 7]. Balloon dilation of the orifice or a ureteral stricture is an option if passage of the ureteroscope is not possible. However, in such cases, we recommend the placement of a ureteral stent which allows passive ureteral dilation, and recommend retrying the insertion after seven to 10 days.

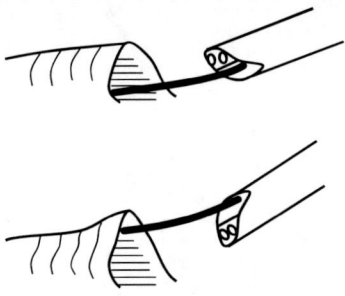

Figure 7.

In order to select an appropriate size of UAS, we usually try inserting an internal obturator of 10 Fr, 12 Fr and 14 Fr in series. If a difficulty is encountered with the insertion, gentle coaxial dilation with the internal obturator may prove useful. However, care should be taken to avoid applying excess sheer force that could lead to ureteral injury or avulsion. If this procedure fails, we place an indwelling ureteral stent, which allows for passive ureteral dilation and successful UAS insertion, after seven to 10 days.

Ureteroscopic access to the lower pole calyx has been challenging. The current flexible ureteroscope can deflect up to 270 degrees, so it can usually reach an acute angle into the lower calyx. However, in cases with severe hydronephrosis, the length of the lower pole infundibulum is sometimes longer than the deflected segment of the ureteroscope. In such cases, lower pole calculi should be repositioned into the upper or middle calyx prior to fragmentation with the Ho:YAG laser. The NGage® basket (Cook), which has an original open-shaped tip, may be helpful in catching the lower calyx stones. In particular, the anterior (ventral) calyx in lower pole is difficult to access. The operator should angle the tip of the ureteroscope and twist it to access the target calyx. When working with a flexible ureteroscope within the kidney, respiratory motion can hinder the laser lithotripsy. In cases under general anesthesia, the anesthesiologist can control the rate and depth of the patient's respiration. However, in the case of spinal anesthesia, especially with sedation, there are sometimes difficulties due to respiratory motion.

When breaking the stone, there are several technical terms, including crush, peel, dig, stick, cut and random shot. The "crush" technique involves compressing or pushing down the stone with the tip of a laser fiber and breaking it into small pieces or a powder [Figure 8a]. The "peel" technique involves removing the outer shell of the large stone, which is relatively easy to break, and then "digging" in the inner hard core of the stone [Figure 8b].

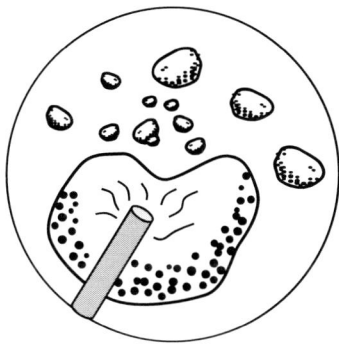

Figure 8a.

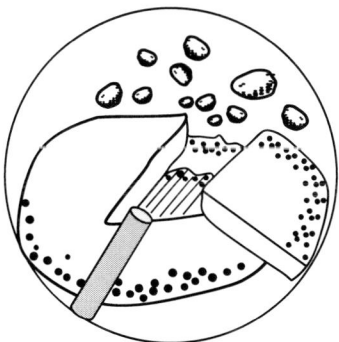

Figure 8b.

The "stick" technique involves piercing the laser fiber into some points of the stone and joining them to break the stone [Figure 8c]. The "cut" technique is associated with shooting the laser linearly in order to cut the stone into appropriately-sized blocks [Figure 8d]. A "random shot" technique can be used to shoot the laser at random in order to comminute small stone fragments in a calyx [Figure 8e].

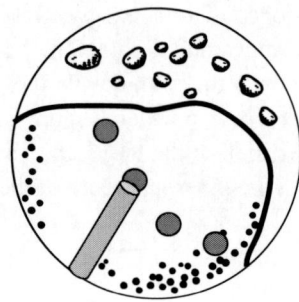

Figure 8c.

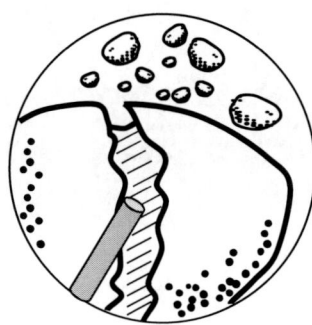

Figure 8d.

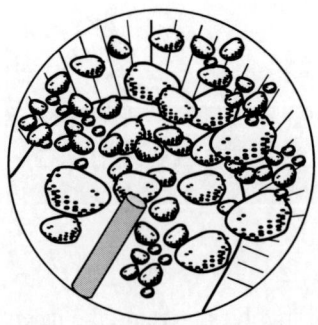

Figure 8e.

If the stone is small enough to extract, it can simply be placed in a basket and removed. When removing the stone fragments, it is necessary to be careful not to cause further damage to the ureter. If any resistance is met, the extraction should be discontinued, because forceful removal may cause critical damage to the ureter. If impaction of the stone is encountered, several options should be considered. First of all, it is necessary to ensure that the guidewire is in placed proximal to the stone. It is the often possible to advance the stone proximally, usually into a more dilated ureteral segment, and then to proceed with further holmium laser lithotripsy. If the stone is lodged within the basket and cannot be extracted, it can be fragmented within the basket. However, if the impacted stone cannot be dislodged, then the basket is extracorporeally disassembled and the ureteroscope is removed, leaving the disassembled basket in place. The ureteroscope is then reintroduced alongside the basket, and the stone within the basket is fragmented, or one of the wires of the basket may be cut off.

The kidney and the upper ureter move with respiration. It is therefore necessary to slow the respiratory movement to stabilize the kidney or at least provide predictable movement. With slow predictable movement, the urologist can anticipate the position of the target as it passes and treat it during that period. The anesthesiologist can usually slow the respiratory rate and decrease the ventilation volume as needed.

Conclusion

In this chapter, we described our routine techniques used for ureteroscopic lithotripsy. We hope that this chapter will be helpful to trainees.

References

[1] Valdivia Uria JG, Valle Gerhold J, Lopez Lopez JA, et al. Technique and complications of percutaneous nephroscopy: experience with 557 patients in the supine position. *J. Urol.* 1998; 160: 1975-8.
[2] Scoffone CM, Cracco CM, Cossu M, et al. Endoscopic combined intrarenal surgery in Galdakao-modified supine Valdivia position: a new standard for percutaneous nephrolithotomy? *Eur. Urol.* 2008; 54: 1393-403.

[3] Hamamoto S, Yasui T, Okada A, et al. Endoscopic combined intrarenal surgery for large calculi: Simultaneous use of flexible ureteroscopy and mini-percutaneous nephrolithotomy overcomes the disadvantageous of percutaneous of percutaneous nephrolithotomy monotherapy. *J. Endourol.* 2014; 28: 28-33.

[4] Yazici CM, Kayhan A, Dogan C. Supine or prone percutaneous nephrolithotomy: Do anatomical changes make it worse? *J. Endourol.* 2014; 28: 10-16.

Chapter 5

Semirigid and Flexible Ureteroscopy: Ohguchi-Higashi Method

Junichi Matsuzaki*, M.D., Ph.D.[1],
Takashi Kawahara, M.D.[1,2,3], Hiroki Ito, M.D.[1,2],
Hiroji Uemura, M.D., Ph.D.[2], Masahiro Yao, M.D., Ph.D.[2]
and Yoshinobu Kubota, M.D., Ph.D.[2]

[1]Department of Urology, Ohguchi Higashi General Hospital, Tokyo, Japan
[2]Department of Urology, Yokohama City University Graduate School of Medicine, Japan
[3]Departments of Pathology and Urology, Johns Hopkins University School of Medicine, Baltimore, Maryland, US

Abstract

The stone treatment with ureteroscopy depends on advances in device. Newer generation flexible ureteroscopes with their greater deflectability, miniaturization and improved tip control are key to the atraumatic inspection of the entire urothelium. In f-URS, ureteral access

---

* Corresponding author: Junichi Matsuzaki, M.D., Ph.D. junmatukd5@yahoo.co.jp.

sheath is the most important parts in the diameter, length and flexibility of the UAS. It is important to use properly the device intraoperatively in many situations. In this chapter, we describe our routine techniques used for ureteroscopic lithotripsy.

Introduction

Over the past 20 years, ureteroscopy (URS) has dramatically changed the management of renal and ureteral calculi. Major technical improvements include endoscope miniaturization, enhanced optical quality and tools, and the introduction of disposables. URS has had a marked impact on active stone removal and is increasingly being performed worldwide.

1. Required Equipment

Fluoroscopic equipment must be available in the operating room. When performing semi-rigid ureteroscopy, a number of items should be considered essential. Typically, all the equipment needed to perform standard rigid cystoscopy is required. Also, when choosing a semi-rigid ureteroscopic approach, we recommend having a variety of guidewires (GW), baskets, ureteral catheters at hand, and in the event that stone management is planned, a holmium YAG (Ho:YAG) laser with 200, 365, or 550 μm fibers should be available (Part 2-1. Instrumentation for ureteroscopic lithotripsy in detail). In cases of flexible ureteroscopy, a ureteral access sheath (UAS) should be used, and in some cases, a UAS may be needed for semi-rigid ureteroscopy.

2. Anesthesia and Position

Distal ureteral stone ureteroscopy is performed under lumbar anesthesia in the lithotomy position, and under general anesthesia for renal stones and proximal and middle ureteral stones. In cases of large stone burden, the procedures will be carried out with the patient in the Galdakao-modified Valdivia position under general anesthesia. The advantages of this position include greater versatility of stone manipulation along the entire upper urinary tract, particularly given the increasing use of retrograde drainage and combined or subsequent retrograde and percutaneous access to the urinary tract with both rigid and flexible instruments [1].

3. Technique

3.1. Rigid Ureteroscopy

Semi-rigid ureteroscopes are routinely used when it can reach the stones. Normally, a semi-rigid ureteroscope can reach the proximal ureter. In some Japanese women, semi-rigid ureteroscopy can reach the renal pelvis and upper calyx. In cases of distal ureteral stones, ureteroscopy is performed without a UAS. In cases of upper and middle ureter stones, insertion of a UAS is preferable because of low intrarenal pressure and treatment efficacy. A semi-rigid ureteroscope with a UAS is useful for treating large stone burden. A flexible ureteroscope should be used when it is difficult to reach stones with a semi-rigid ureteroscope.

6/7.5-Fr semi-rigid ureteroscopes (Wolf, Knittlingen, Germany) are routinely used. For proximal and distal ureteral stones, a semi-rigid ureteroscope is introduced into the ureter with a safety wire in place. After confirming the correct side and performing cystoscopic examination of the bladder, a GW is placed into the ureteral orifice and its position is confirmed by fluoroscopy. We recommend, whenever possible, that semi-rigid ureteroscopy be performed alongside a stiff wire, such as a Tornado™ (Piolax, Yokohama Japan).

Endourologists should always have a laterolateral image of the course of the viscera that highlights the relatively accentuated and focused angle that the ureter takes when bypassing the iliac vessels, bringing it directly into the bladder. A full understanding of the ureteroscopic route inside each individual tract of the ureter will almost always help avoid traumatic injury.

Another anatomical consideration to bear in mind is the structure: the delicate mucosa, the muscular layer, and the adventitial layer. The muscular layer, in particular, has different levels of thickness from the top (thinner) to the bottom (thicker), thus making incomplete perforations with a submucosal tunnel in the distal tract, and avulsions or complete perforations in the proximal tract, more frequent. The hydrophilic floppy tip of the GW facilitates passage beyond obstructions and negotiates tortuous anatomy.

At this point, the GW tip should be under the level of the iliac crest because the coiling GW in the renal pelvis causes mucosal bleeding. After the scope passes the ureteral orifice, the GW is pulled out from the end of the scope. This technique decreases mucosal damage by the GW because the GW rarely migrates under the ureteral mucosa.

If resistance is noted when advancing the endoscope, retrograde ureteropyelography shows kinking of the ureter or stricture. The procedure can continue if there only is slight resistance and a ureteral stent should be inserted in this case at the end of the procedure. If severe stricture of the ureter is encountered, the procedure should be stopped and ureteroscopy can be performed without resistance 1–2 weeks later.

3.2. Intra-Ureteral Lithotripsy

The most effective lithotripsy system is the Ho:YAG laser, which has become the gold standard for ureteroscopy, because it is effective for all stone types [2–4]. Pneumatic and ultrasound systems can be used with high disintegration efficacy in rigid URS [5–7]. However, stone migration into the kidney is a common problem, which can be prevented by placing special tools proximal to the stone [8]. In semi-rigid ureteroscopy, the UAS should be inserted up to the edge of the stone as this position is ideal for appropriate irrigation flow. The stones are then fragmented using a 550-μm fiber laser with basic energy and frequency settings of 0.5–1.0 J and 5–10 Hz (2.5–10 W), respectively. However, in some cases of hard stones (e.g., oxalate monohydrate or cystine stones), the energy should be increased to 1.5–2.5 J. The settings should be changed during the procedure based on the lithotripsy effects. The criteria for terminating laser lithotripsy are complete fragment extraction of the ureter stones or residual fragments <1 mm with the expectation of spontaneous excretion [9]. Misfiring to the mucosa may cause ureteral stricture, so the tip of the laser should be placed on the mucosa. In cases of an impacted stone attached to the ureteral wall, the stone is fragmented into a floating state and the fragments are removed with a basket catheter. The operator holds and manipulates the basket catheter with an endoscope. After completing semi-rigid ureteroscopy, the GW is inserted and the flexible ureteroscope is inserted along the GW. It is necessary to ensure there are no residual fragments in the upper urinary tract under fluoroscopic and visual guidance. If residual fragments are observed, a flexible ureteroscope should be inserted with a UAS. If there are no residual fragments, the GW should be inserted and the ureteroscope retracted over the GW under visual guidance.

3.3. Flexible Ureteroscopy

Minimally invasive surgery is preferable for patients with renal stones because of excellent stone clearance and low morbidity. Major technological progress has been achieved in retrograde intrarenal surgery, with improved deflection mechanisms and durability [10–12]. Initial experience with digital scopes has demonstrated shorter operation times due to improvements in image quality [13–15]. A flexible URS is used mainly for the renal collecting system and, in cases with difficult anatomy, the upper ureter.

The problem of lower-pole access has been addressed by examining the deflection properties of flexible ureteroscopes. Major problems with the flexible ureteroscopes currently available are their high maintenance costs and time lost when the scope needs repair or replacement. Therefore, it is very important to take care of flexible ureteroscopes: they are to be used as linearized as possible and without excessive force.

3.4. Ureteral Access Sheath

A hydrophilic-coated UAS, which is available in different calibers (inner diameter ≥9.5 F), can be inserted via a GW, with the tip placed in the proximal ureter. UAS allows easy and multiple access to the upper urinary tract and therefore significantly facilitates URS. The use of UAS improves vision by establishing a continuous outflow, decreasing intrarenal pressure, and potentially reducing operation time [16, 17]. It also allows for repeated and rapid passage of a flexible ureteroscope during upper urinary tract endourologic procedures. Insertion of a UAS may lead to ureteral damage; however, no data on long-term consequences are available [18]. It is better to use a UAS of smaller diameter at the point of ureteral ischemia. The UAS diameter will be determined by preoperative stenting and rigid ureteroscopy findings. Generally, in cases of an indwelling preoperative stent, a UAS of 13/15 Fr or 14/16 Fr can be inserted. In cases without a preoperative stent, a UAS of 11/13 Fr or 12/14 Fr can be inserted. In Japanese men, it is preferable to select a 45-cm UAS for kidney stones and a 35-cm UAS for upper ureteral stones. In woman, a 35-cm UAS should be used for both types of stones. The

UAS should be gently inserted over the GW under fluoroscopy. If resistance is encountered when inserting the UAS, it should be carefully removed in a single movement leaving only the inner tube to dilate the ureter. If additional resistance is encountered when inserting the inner tube, a ureteral stent (6–8 Fr) should be inserted, and the procedure should be delayed for 1 or 2 weeks. For lithotomy of a stone <5 mm, ureteroscopy can be done without a UAS. The UAS is inserted up to 5 cm before the stones while considering the length of the bending section of the flexible scope. In cases of kidney stones, the UAS is usually placed in front of the ureteropelvic junction. In cases of upper calyceal or renal pelvic stones, it is also effective if the tip of the UAS is inserted up to the renal pelvis and upper calyx. In cases of middle and lower pole stones, the same technique can be applied after repositioning the upper calyx. After inserting the ureteroscope, sufficient irrigation flow should be verified. Nevertheless, with a poor field of view at the renal pelvis, repetitive suction and injection can improve vision for excluding dust-like debris through the ureteroscope port. With the UAS in the proper position, the irrigation flow in the kidney can be confirmed by observing the irrigation fluid, which flows continuously through the ureteroscope channel and out through the UAS. In cases of poor irrigation, it is necessary to change the position of the UAS. Without sufficient irrigation, ureteroscopic lithotomy for urolithiasis should be avoided and ureteral stents should be inserted to dilate the ureter and the procedure delayed. Adequate flow during the procedure is important during laser lithotripsy as it helps keep a clear field of view for the surgeon to visualize the target. To control expansion of the renal pelvis intraoperatively, it is important to change the position of the top edge of the UAS appropriately during the procedure. In cases of caudal insertion of the UAS tip, strong hydronephrosis makes repositioning of stones easy, but a risk of postoperative infection increases due to the increase in intrarenal pressure. In cases of cranial insertion, slight hydronephrosis makes it difficult to orientate the scope in the renal pelvis.

To maintain a clear ureteroscopic view, the irrigant is pumped manually and intermittently during the procedure. This pumping consists of intermittent or continuous press and suction.

3.5. Extraction

The aim of URS is complete stone removal, especially ureteral stones. Stones or stone fragments are extracted from the kidney through the access sheath of the ureteroscope using baskets. Nitinol (nickel-titanium alloy) baskets provide additional advantages over steel wire baskets, such as increased flexibility. Tipless versions of nitinol baskets are also available for use in calices. The basket catheter has two roles. One is extracting stones <1 mm in size. It is efficient to retrieve as large stones as possible to decrease operation time. The other role is stone displacement. Stones >5 mm should be displaced into the upper calyx or renal pelvis with the help of a basket and fragmented with the Ho: YAG laser. This step helps increase the life of the flexible ureteroscope. Small stones are basketed out with a (1.5 Fr Cook) N-Circle basket. If a calyceal stone is too big to be basketable, it is fragmented into two or three pieces by the laser. The fragments are then repositioned into the upper calyx where they are fragmented with the Ho:YAG laser. There is no evidence that fragments of all sizes should be removed for uneventful postoperative observation. We try to remove 0.5–1 mm fragments as much as possible to prevent recurrence of urolithiasis.

3.6. Intra-Renal Lithotripsy

The Ho: YAG laser is also effective in flexible ureteroscopy. For lithotripsy, 200-μm lasers are the first choice because of their small influence on scope deflection. Laser lithotripsy is performed in situ, without displacement of the stone from the lower pole. Stone displacement prior to fragmentation is associated with a higher stone-free rate compared with patients who undergo in situ fragmentation. The fragments repositioned into the upper calyx are fragmented with a 365-μm fiber laser. Placing an instrument through a flexible ureteroscope impedes scope deflection, which may make it difficult or impossible to perform laser lithotripsy of lower pole calculi.

Power setting: Energy and frequency settings for a 3–10 W laser are 0.5–1.0 J and 5–10 Hz, respectively. The criteria for terminating laser lithotripsy are complete fragment extraction or residual fragments <2 mm and the expectation of spontaneous excretion. Ideal lithotripsy is fragmentation to the maximum size of the stone that can be passed through a UAS.

Three methods are used to fragment stones:

- Vaporization method: The fiber laser is moved over the stone just like painting with a brush; this method is used in the case of soft stones.

- Fragmentation method: The stone is drilled multiple times and the intermittent ridge is fragmented into small pieces in the case of hard stones.
- Popcorn effect: This method is used to break large fragments into tiny pieces; the laser is fired in the middle of the large fragments from a distance of about 5 mm without focusing on any particular fragment. The energy is not changed, but the frequency is increased to 15–25 Hz. This causes the fragments to fly like popcorn and in the process the stones are hit by the fiber laser, which fragments them. This method helps create fragments small enough to be passed in the urine. In addition, much time is saved compared with breaking down individual fragments. Free-flying fragments in the irrigation fluid indicate that the fragments are sufficiently small to be passed in the urine.

4. Tips and Tricks

Fluoroscopic equipment must be available in the operating room. A safety GW is not placed routinely, even though some groups removing an impacted stone have demonstrated that URS should be performed with a GW [19, 20]. A safety wire prevents false passage in cases of perforation and ensures that a double J stent can be inserted in difficult situations, thus avoiding significant complications. The residual fragment is checked under fluoroscopic and visual guidance. Under fluoroscopy, radiation is continuously emitted while rotating the C-arm.

5. Postoperative Stenting

A ureteral stent should be inserted in the case of ureteral stricture and impacted stones. Insertion of a postoperative ureteral stent should be avoided where possible. If ureteropyelography at the end of the procedure shows good urine flow in the ureter, postoperative double J stenting can be omitted, and the externalized ureteral catheter can be placed in one night. For stones <1 cm with no impaction, a procedure without a ureteral stent can be done in over 50% of cases. Stentless URS with an externalized ureteral catheter is as feasible as double J stenting. Moreover, stent-related discomforts due to the presence of a double J stent and the need for postoperative cystoscopy to remove the stent can be avoided with an externalized ureteral catheter [21].

Conclusion

Semirigid and flexible ureteroscopy is key component of urologic practice today. It is important to use properly the device, example for ueterosope, laser setting, ureteral access sheath and basket catheter.

References

[1] Ibarluzea G, Scoffone CM, Cracco CM, et al. Supine Valdivia and modified lithotomy position for simultaneous anterograde and retrograde endourological access. *BJU Int.* 2007; 100: 233-6.

[2] Leijte JA, Oddens JR, Lock TM. Holmium laser lithotripsy for ureteral calculi: predictive factors for complications and success. *J. Endourol.* 2008; 22:257-60.

[3] Marguet CG, Sung JC, Springhart WP, et al. In vitro comparison of stone retropulsion and fragmentation of the frequency doubled, double pulse nd:yag laser and the holmium:yag laser. *J. Urol.* 2005; 173: 1797-800.

[4] Pierre S, Preminger GM. Holmium laser for stone management. *World J. Urol.* 2007; 25: 235-9.

[5] Garg S, Mandal AK, Singh SK, et al. Ureteroscopic laser lithotripsy versus ballistic lithotripsy for treatment of ureteric stones: a prospective comparative study. *Urol. Int.* 2009; 82: 341-5.

[6] Vorreuther R, Klotz T, Heidenreich A, et al. Pneumatic v electrokinetic lithotripsy in treatment of ureteral stones. *J. Endourol.* 1998; 12: 233-6.

[7] Binbay M, Tepeler A, Singh A, et al. Evaluation of pneumatic versus holmium:YAG laser lithotripsy for impacted ureteral stones. *Int. Urol. Nephrol.* 2011; 43: 989-95.

[8] Ahmed M, Pedro RN, Kieley S, et al. Systematic evaluation of ureteral occlusion devices: insertion, deployment, stone migration, and extraction. *Urology.* 2009; 73: 976-80.

[9] Seitz C, Tanovic E, Kikic Z, et al. Impact of stone size, location, composition, impaction, and hydronephrosis on the efficacy of holmium:YAG-laser ureterolithotripsy. *Eur. Urol.* 2007; 52: 1751-7.

[10] Wendt-Nordahl G, Mut T, Krombach P, et al. Do new generation flexible ureterorenoscopes offer a higher treatment success than their predecessors? *Urol. Res.* 2011; 39: 185-8.

[11] Knudsen B, Miyaoka R, Shah K, et al. Durability of the next-generation flexible fiberoptic ureteroscopes: a randomized prospective multi-institutional clinical trial. *Urology.* 2010; 75: 534-8.

[12] Skolarikos AA, Papatsoris AG, Mitsogiannis IC, et al. Current status of ureteroscopic treatment for urolithiasis. *Int. J. Urol.* 2009; 16: 713-7.

[13] Binbay M, Yuruk E, Akman T, et al. Is there a difference in outcomes between digital and fiberoptic flexible ureterorenoscopy procedures? *J. Endourol.* 2010; 24: 1929-34.

[14] Humphreys MR, Miller NL, Williams JC Jr, et al. A new world revealed: early experience with digital ureteroscopy. *J. Urol.* 2008; 179: 970-5.

[15] Mitchell S, Havranek E, Patel A. First digital flexible ureterorenoscope: initial experience. *J. Endourol.* 2008; 22: 47-50.

[16] Stern JM, Yiee J, Park S. Safety and efficacy of ureteral access sheaths. *J. Endourol.* 2007; 21: 119-23.

[17] L'esperance JO, Ekeruo WO, Scales CD Jr, et al. Effect of ureteral access sheath on stone-free rates in patients undergoing ureteroscopic management of renal calculi. *Urology.* 2005; 66: 252-5.

[18] Traxer O, Thomas A. Prospective evaluation and classification of ureteral wall injuries resulting from insertion of a ureteral access sheath during retrograde intrarenal surgery. *J. Urol.* 2013; 189: 580-4.

[19] Dickstein RJ, Kreshover JE, Babayan RK, et al. Is a safety wire necessary during routine flexible ureteroscopy? *J. Endourol.* 2010; 24: 1589-92.

[20] Eandi JA, Hu B, Low RK. Evaluation of the impact and need for use of a safety guidewire during ureteroscopy. *J. Endourol.* 2008; 22: 1653-8.

[21] Kawahara T, Ito H, Terao H, et al. Early ureteral catheter removal after ureteroscopic lithotripsy using ureteral access sheath. *Urolithiasis.* 2013; 41: 31-5.

Chapter 6

Stenting and Postoperative Care

Takashi Kawahara[*], M.D.[1,2,3], Hiroki Ito, M.D.[1,2],
Hiroji Uemura, M.D., Ph.D.[2],
Yoshinobu Kubota, M.D., Ph.D.[2]
and Junichi Matsuzaki, M.D., Ph.D.[1]*

[1]Department of Urology, Ohguchi Higashi General Hospital, Japan
[2]Department of Urology, Yokohama City University
Graduate School of Medicine, Japan
[3]Departments of Pathology and Urology,
Johns Hopkins University School of Medicine, Baltimore, Maryland, US

Abstract

The development of flexible ureteroscopy (URS) has allowed for a variety of ureteral procedures to be successfully performed. In addition, there are several endoscopic procedures, including rigid and flexible URS, ureteral access sheaths (UAS), ureteral stents, basket devices for retrieving stone fragments and many types of lasers. The use of ureteral stents was first reported by Zimskind et al. in 1967. Since then, these stents have been become essential for maintaining ureteral patency during various types of endoscopic procedures. This chapter describes our experience with the endoscopic management of postoperative ureteral stents.

---

[*] Corresponding author: Takashi Kawahara, M.D. takashi_tk2001@yahoo.co.jp.

Introduction

Ureteroscopy (URS) is frequently used with a high rate of success in the management of ureteral stones [1-3]. Following the development of flexible URS, Ho: YAG laser lithotripsy and basket devices to retrieve stone fragments, the ureteral access sheath (UAS) has become an essential tool in the treatment of renal stones [3, 4]. However, the use of UAS carries a potential risk of ureteral stenosis due to ureteral mucosal ischemia with subsequent mucosal edema causing hydronephrosis [5]. The purpose of postoperative ureteral stenting is to prevent ureteral stricture and reduce the incidence of postoperative renal colic [1, 6, 7]. Ureteral stenting also contributes to the passage of small stone fragments due to ureteral edema [6, 8-12]. In this chapter, we describe postoperative ureteral catheterization.

1. Reducing Ureteral Stent-Related Symptoms

1.1. Types of Ureteral Stents

Ureteral stents contain various materials and are available in different sizes, coatings and shapes in order to prevent unpleasant urinary symptoms and discomfort [13-15]. It is necessary to minimize the amount of material in the bladder in order to decrease the incidence of stent-related symptoms [13]. Therefore, the Tail Stent® (Boston Scientific, USA) was developed with a 7-Fr proximal pigtail at the proximal end and a 7-Fr shaft that tapers to a lumenless straight 3-Fr tail at the distal end [16]. Dunn et al. showed that the use of 7-Fr tail loop stents produces significantly less irritating symptoms than that associated with standard 7-Fr double-pigtail stents. Lingeman et al. evaluated stent-related symptoms associated with various types of ureteral stents using a self-administered questionnaire and found that the use of loop-type ureteral stents resulted in lower stent-related symptom scores than those observed in the patients treated with standard double stents, although the difference was not significant [17]. We investigated the effectiveness of changing to loop-type ureteral stents among a total of 25 patients with a median age of 56.5 years (52.9 ± 12.2 years) treated with ureteral stent exchange [18]. The incidence of almost all stent-related symptoms, except nocturia, was significantly lower among the patients treated with loop-type ureteral stents than among those treated with double pigtail stents. With respect to the ureteral stent position, the symptom scores were differentiated according to a stent location at the distal end. When the shaft of the stent was placed across the midline, the symptom scores were higher than those observed when the shaft was placed fully inside the ureter. Therefore, it is necessary to select the appropriate length of ureteral stent, and changing to the loop-type ureteral stent significantly decreases the incidence of ureteral stent-related symptoms.

1.2. Length of Ureteral Stents

Changing to loop-type ureteral stents significantly decreases the incidence of ureteral stent-related symptoms [18]. However, inserting an inappropriate length of ureteral stent is pointless. Therefore, choosing the optimal length of the ureteral stent is important for decreasing the incidence of stent migration and other complications [19-24]. We investigated the correlation between ureteral length and the ureteral stent length among patients treated with 226 loop-type ureteral stents using direct ureteral length measurements. Nine stents (3.9%) were found to have migrated, while 171 stents (75.7%) were found to be in the appropriate position and 46 stents (19.5%) were found to be too long. In this study, we placed ureteral stents that were the same length as the ureter; however, 10 of 91 stents (11.0%) were found to be longer than the ureter when the proximal ureteral stent was placed in the renal pelvis. Obtaining direct measurements using ureteral catheters is thought to be the optimal method for choosing the appropriate length of the ureteral stent. The appropriate length of the ureteral stent is the same or 1 cm less than the measured ureteral length. The use of ureteral stents more than 2 cm smaller than the measured ureteral length is associated with an increasing incidence of migration. Employing ureteral stents measuring 1 cm shorter than the ureteral length is ideal, with a 2.6% risk of migration and an 8.6% risk of being too long.

Choosing a ureteral stent based on direct ureteral length measurements is ideal, although both the patient and operator are exposed to additional radiation and an extra procedure is required. Therefore, it is necessary to estimate the ureteral length. The correlation with the patient's height is generally used to estimate the ureteral length. However, the reliability of this method has not yet been confirmed [25]. A variety of methods for estimating the actual ureteral length (AUL) have been reported, including: (1) assessing the patient's body height, (2) measuring variables of body habitus, (3) obtaining direct measurements of the ureter using a ureteral catheter, (4) obtaining direct measurements using a guidewire, (5) performing ureteral tracing via intravenous urography (IVU), (6) measuring the distance from the ureteropelvic junction (UPJ) to the ureterovesical junction (UVJ) on IVU and (7) measuring the distance from the mid kidney to the UVJ on IVU [26-29]. We analyzed patients who underwent both preoperative IVU and CT. The ureteral length was measured in 151 Japanese patients (94 males, 57 females, 169 ureters) using a ruled 5-Fr ureteral catheter (TigerTail®, BARD, USA). We assessed the correlations between the actual ureteral length and (1) body height (BH), (2) body surface area (BSA), (3) ureteral trace (UT) on IVU, (4) the linear distance (Linear Distance 1: LD1) from the UPJ to the UVJ on IVU, (5) the linear distance (Linear Distance 2: LD2) from the mid kidney to the UVJ on IVU and (6) the distance from the level of the renal vein to UVJ on non-contrast axial computed tomography (CT) (axial CT distance: ACTD). The correlation coefficients for BH, BSA, UT, LD1, LD2 and ACTD were 0.3258, 0.3255, 0.4917, 0.5413, 0.5265 and 0.6124, respectively. The ACTD was found to correlate best with the actual ureteral length, as predicted by the Spearman correlation coefficient. The AUL was calculated for each variable: BH-AUL (cm): 0.0687 x BH (cm) + 12.05. BSA-AUL (cm): 3.3167 x BSA (m^2) + 17.69. UT-AUL (cm): 0.3739 x UT (cm) + 13.94. LD1-AUL (cm): 0.398 x LD1 (cm) + 13.71. LD2-AUL (cm): 0.4134 x LD2 (cm) + 12.56. ACTD-AUL (cm): 0.044 x ACTD (mm) + 13.25. The ACTD was therefore found to predict the actual ureteral length better than BH, BSA or IVU, while the ACTD was found to be a reliable predictor of the ureteral length. Therefore, obtaining direct ureteral length measurements is ideal, although measuring the ACTD is a new option for estimating the ureteral length and subsequently choosing the appropriate length of ureteral stent.

1.3. Duration of Ureteral Stenting

Serious complications, including migration, fragmentation and stone formation, can occur, particularly when stents have been forgotten after a long period [30-33]. However, no widespread guidelines exist for the management of these potentially serious problems [34]. The mechanism underlying the development of encrustation in patients with infected urine involves the presence of organic components in the urine crystallizing onto the surface of the biomaterial and subsequently being incorporated into a bacterial biofilm layer. The bacteria continue to grow, resulting in the production of urease, which attacks urea, thereby increasing the urinary pH. The increased pH attracts calcium and magnesium ions to the biofilm matrix, which results in crystal formation [35, 36]. The incidence of encrustation has been shown to increase in association with the duration of the placement of an indwelling stent [37]. We investigated the correlation between the indwelling time and the development of encrustation, coloration and resistance to removal in 330 involving of ureteral stents. A total of 181 patients underwent removal of 330 internal ureteral stents: 324 (98.2%) stents for stone disease and six (1.8%) stents for benign ureteral stricture. Of these patients, 50 underwent two replacement procedures, 23 underwent three replacement procedures, six underwent four replacement procedures, three underwent five replacement procedures and one underwent seven replacement procedures in each site. Overall, 155 stents (47.0%) were found to be encrusted. The stent length and patency (encrustation, coloration and resistance to removal) were not found to be significantly correlated. In terms of the stent caliber, the use of stents measuring less than 6-Fr in size was associated with a significantly higher rate of encrustation than that observed in the patients treated with stents measuring over 7-Fr in size. The frequency of encrustation with coloration was higher than that without coloration among the patients treated with indwelling stents for a period of less of six weeks and or six to 12 weeks. A report by el-Faqih et al. indicated that the rate of stent encrustation increases from 9.2% following an indwelling time of less than six weeks to 47.5% at six to 12 weeks to 76.3% at more than 12 weeks [37]. Our observations support these data, as the rate of stent encrustation was 26.8% at less than six weeks, 56.9% at six to 12 weeks and 75.9% at more than 12 weeks in the present study. Our study included a total of 33 patients who had undergone the insertion of two or more stents on the same side. Among patients with stents exhibiting encrustation, we therefore suggest that the ureteral stent be exchanged sooner than the initial indwelling time in order to avoid encrustation. As a result of following this recommendation, the encrustation rate for the initial insertion was 64.2% (median indwelling time: 62 days) and that for the second insertion was 41.8% (median indwelling time: 45 days) in the same patient group (p=0.01). In our study, although the development of ureteral stent encrustation was related to the indwelling time, heavily encrusted ureteral stents that required additional procedures for removal (SWL and/or URS) were detected within three months of implantation. The optimal interval for removing an indwelling ureteral stent to avoid additional procedures is difficult to determine and is likely both patient- and situation-dependent. We employed the Kaplan Meier method (with encrustation as the endpoint instead of death) and found a 60% survival (non-encrustation) rate at 60 days and a 30% survival rate at 90-100 days of indwelling time. In our hospital, ureteral stent replacement is recommended within three months in order to prevent heavy encrustation and urosepsis.

2. Decreasing the Invasiveness of Ureteral Stent Removal

The use of ureteral stents was first reported by Zimskind et al. in 1967. Subsequently, ureteral stents have become essential for maintaining ureteral patency in patients treated with postoperative ureteroscopic procedures. However, serious complications, including migration, fragmentation and stone formation, can still occur, particularly when the stent has been forgotten after a long period [30-33].

The incidence of encrustation increases in association with the duration of indwelling stent placement [37, 38]. Therefore, stents require periodic replacement or removal. The standard technique used to remove a ureteral stent involves cystoscopy [39, 40].

Cystoscopy is a fundamental urologic procedure; however, inserting a cystoscope is invasive. We developed a method for removing ureteral stents in female patients using a crochet hook that requires no cystoscopy or fluoroscopic guidance [41] [42]. Crochet hooks are used to knit fabric and knit patterns from yarn, such as sweaters.

A crochet hook made of metal was selected and sterilized via autoclaving. Lidocaine gel (2%) was spread on the hook, which was then inserted into the urethra. The crochet hook was advanced toward ureteral orifice and carefully passed to the urethra and over the bladder mucosa. The detailed technique was presented in our previous report [41].

In that study, 47 of 54 stents were successfully removed (87.0%). The mean visual analogue pain scale was 1.5 for stent removal using a crochet hook and 3.0 for stent removal using cystoscopy ($p<0.05$). Therefore, performing ureteral stent removal using a crochet hook is easy, safe and cost effective. This technique is also easy to learn and is therefore considered to be suitable for use in outpatient clinics.

3. One Night Catheters

We previously reported the new option of using one night ureteral catheterization following ureteroscopic lithotripsy with UAS [5]. A total of 63 patients were treated at the conclusion of URS one day after the operation. The presence of hydronephrosis was assessed three days after URS using US and the presence of residual stones was checked two weeks after URS using CT. The early removal of the ureteral catheter was associated with a correlation between the operative time and the incidence of hydronephrosis. Hydronephrosis was detected on US three days after URS in 34 patients (54.0%) and on CT two weeks after URS in four patients (6.3%). Among these four patients, no hydronephrosis was observed during two months of follow-up. With respect to the operative time, the hydronephrosis group (three days after URS) exhibited a significantly higher operative time (mean: 58.9 min., median: 53 min.) than the non-hydronephrosis group (mean: 45.5 min., median: 43 min.). (p=0.03) No patients visited the emergency room due to intolerable pain. In this study, we set the protocol to include early removal of the ureteral catheter, not stentless URS after ureteroscopic lithotripsy. The most important point when performing stentless URS is to decrease urinary symptoms without requiring additional ureteral stent removal using cystoscopy in a safe clinical manner after URS. We rarely encountered patients with severely edematous ureters and ureteral orifices after URS, in whom we were unable to insert a guidewire into the ureter; therefore, additional procedures for performing percutaneous nephrostomy must be developed. We believe that, in most cases, stentless URS can be performed safely, although critical cases should be treated with ureteral stent reinsertion. Therefore, one night ureteral catheterization provides the security of successful ureteral stent reinsertion. In addition, one night ureteral catheterization is less painful and associated with lower costs than double pigtail ureteral stenting due to the lack of need for cystoscopy during removal. Therefore, one night ureteral catheterization is a potential new option for providing postoperative care, in particular among patients who receive ureteroscopic lithotripsy for approximately 50 minutes.

Conclusion

The early removal of ureteral catheters can be safely performed in patients who undergo URS with UAS, except for those with a potential risk for the development of ureteral stricture, including subjects with impacted stones, preoperative ureteral stricture, intraoperative ureteral injury and/or a longer operative time.

References

[1] Chen YT, Chen J, Wong WY, Yang SS, Hsieh CH, Wang CC: Is ureteral stenting necessary after uncomplicated ureteroscopic lithotripsy? A prospective, randomized controlled trial. *J. Urol.* 2002; 167: 1977-80.
[2] Kawahara T, Ito H, Terao H, Ishigaki H, Ogawa T, Uemura H, Kubota Y, Matsuzaki J: Preoperative stenting for ureteroscopic lithotripsy for a large renal stone. *Int. J. Urol.* 2012; 19: 881-5..
[3] Ito H, Kawahara T, Terao H, Ogawa T, Yao M, Kubota Y, Matsuzaki J: Predictive Value of Attenuation Coefficients Measured as Hounsfield Units on Noncontrast Computed Tomography During Flexible Ureteroscopy with Holmium Laser Lithotripsy: A Single-Center Experience. *J. Endourol.* 2012; 26: 1125-30.
[4] Ito H, Kawahara T, Terao H, Ogawa T, Yao M, Kubota Y, Matsuzaki J: The Most Reliable Preoperative Assessment of Renal Stone Burden as a Predictor of Stone-free Status After Flexible Ureteroscopy With Holmium Laser Lithotripsy: A Single-center Experience. *Urology.* 2012; 80: 524-8.
[5] Kawahara T, Ito H, Terao H, Kakizoe M, Kato Y, Uemura H, Kubota Y, Matsuzaki J: Early ureteral catheter removal after ureteroscopic lithotripsy using ureteral access sheath. *Urolithiasis.* 2013; 41: 31-5.
[6] Harmon WJ, Sershon PD, Blute ML, Patterson DE, Segura JW: Ureteroscopy: current practice and long-term complications. *J. Urol.* 1997; 157: 28-32.
[7] Netto Junior NR, Claro Jde A, Esteves SC, Andrade EF: Ureteroscopic stone removal in the distal ureter. Why change? *J. Urol.* 1997; 157: 2081-3.
[8] Borboroglu PG, Amling CL, Schenkman NS, Monga M, Ward JF, Piper NY, Bishoff JT, Kane CJ: Ureteral stenting after ureteroscopy for distal ureteral calculi: a multi-institutional prospective randomized controlled study assessing pain, outcomes and complications. *J. Urol.* 2001; 166: 1651-57.

[9] Boddy SA, Nimmon CC, Jones S, Ramsay JW, Britton KE, Levison DA, Whitifield HN: Acute ureteric dilatation for ureteroscopy. An experimental study. *Br. J. Urol.* 1988; 61: 27-31.
[10] Weinberg JJ, Snyder JA, Smith AD: Mechanical extraction of stones with rigid ureteroscopes. *Urol. Clin. North. Am.* 1988; 15: 339-46.
[11] Leventhal EK, Rozanski TA, Crain TW, Deshon GE, Jr.: Indwelling ureteral stents as definitive therapy for distal ureteral calculi. *J. Urol.* 1995; 153: 34-6.
[12] Deliveliotis C, Giannakopoulos S, Louras G, Koutsokalis G, Alivizatos G, Kostakopoulos A: Double-pigtail stents for distal ureteral calculi: an alternative form of definitive treatment. *Urol. Int.* 1996; 57: 224-6.
[13] Lingeman JE, Preminger GM, Goldfischer ER, Krambeck AE: Assessing the impact of ureteral stent design on patient comfort. *J. Urol.* 2009; 181: 2581-7.
[14] Joshi HB, Chitale SV, Nagarajan M, Irving SO, Browning AJ, Biyani CS, Burgess NA: A prospective randomized single-blind comparison of ureteral stents composed of firm and soft polymer. *J. Urol.* 2005; 174: 2303-6.
[15] Dellis A, Joshi HB, Timoney AG, Keeley FX, Jr.: Relief of stent related symptoms: review of engineering and pharmacological solutions. *J. Urol.* 2010; 184: 1267-72.
[16] Dunn MD, Portis AJ, Kahn SA, Yan Y, Shalhav AL, Elbahnasy AM, Bercowsky E, Hoenig DM, Wolf JS, Jr., McDougall EM et al: Clinical effectiveness of new stent design: randomized single-blind comparison of tail and double-pigtail stents. *J. Endourol.* 2000; 14: 195-202.
[17] Lingeman JE, Preminger GM, Goldfischer ER, Krambeck AE: Assessing the impact of ureteral stent design on patient comfort. *J. Urol.* 2009; 181: 2581-7.
[18] Kawahara T, Ito H, Terao H, Ogawa T, Uemura H, Kubota Y, Matsuzaki J: Changing to a loop-type ureteral stent decreases patients' stent-related symptoms. *Urologic. Res.* 2012; 40: 763-767.
[19] Wills MI, Gilbert HW, Chadwick DJ, Harrison SC: Which ureteric stent length? *Br. J. Urol.* 1991; 68: 440.
[20] Pocock RD, Stower MJ, Ferro MA, Smith PJ, Gingell JC: Double J stents. A review of 100 patients. *Br. J. Urol.* 1986; 58: 629-33.
[21] Chin JL, Denstedt JD: Retrieval of proximally migrated ureteral stents. *J. Urol.* 1992; 148: 1205-6.
[22] Slaton JW, Kropp KA: Proximal ureteral stent migration: an avoidable complication? *J. Urol.* 1996; 155: 58-61.

[23] Kawahara T, Ito H, Terao H, Yoshida M, Ogawa T, Uemura H, Kubota Y, Matsuzaki J: Choosing an appropriate length of loop type ureteral stent using direct ureteral length measurement. *Urol. Int.* 2012; 88: 48-53.

[24] Kawahara T, Ito H, Terao H, Yoshida M, Ogawa T, Uemura H, Kubota Y, Matsuzaki J: Which is the best method to estimate the actual ureteral length in patients undergoing ureteral stent placement? *Int. J. Urol.* 2012; 19: 634-8.

[25] Shah J, Kulkarni RP: Height does not predict ureteric length. *Clin. Radiol.* 2005; 60: 812-4.

[26] Pilcher JM, Patel U: Choosing the correct length of ureteric stent: a formula based on the patient's height compared with direct ureteric measurement. *Clin. Radiol.* 2002; 57: 59-62.

[27] Paick SH, Park HK, Byun SS, Oh SJ, Kim HH: Direct ureteric length measurement from intravenous pyelography: does height represent ureteric length? *Urol. Res.* 2005; 33: 199-202.

[28] Hruby GW, Ames CD, Yan Y, Monga M, Landman J: Correlation of ureteric length with anthropometric variables of surface body habitus. *BJU. Int.* 2007; 99: 1119-22.

[29] Ho CH, Huang KH, Chen SC, Pu YS, Liu SP, Yu HJ: Choosing the ideal length of a double-pigtail ureteral stent according to body height: study based on a Chinese population. *Urol. Int.* 2009; 83: 70-4.

[30] Bultitude MF, Tiptaft RC, Glass JM, Dasgupta P: Management of encrusted ureteral stents impacted in upper tract. *Urology.* 2003; 62: 622-6.

[31] Borboroglu PG, Kane CJ: Current management of severely encrusted ureteral stents with a large associated stone burden. *J. Urol.* 2000; 164: 648-50.

[32] Mohan-Pillai K, Keeley FX, Jr., Moussa SA, Smith G, Tolley DA: Endourological management of severely encrusted ureteral stents. *J. Endourol.* 1999; 13: 377-9.

[33] Schulze KA, Wettlaufer JN, Oldani G: Encrustation and stone formation: complication of indwelling ureteral stents. *Urology.* 1985; 25: 616-9.

[34] Singh I, Gupta NP, Hemal AK, Aron M, Seth A, Dogra PN: Severely encrusted polyurethane ureteral stents: management and analysis of potential risk factors. *Urology.* 2001; 58: 526-31.

[35] Keane PF, Bonner MC, Johnston SR, Zafar A, Gorman SP: Characterization of biofilm and encrustation on ureteric stents in vivo. *Br. J. Urol.* 1994; 73: 687-91.
[36] Wollin TA, Tieszer C, Riddell JV, Denstedt JD, Reid G: Bacterial biofilm formation, encrustation, and antibiotic adsorption to ureteral stents indwelling in humans. *J. Endourol.* 1998; 12: 101-11.
[37] el-Faqih SR, Shamsuddin AB, Chakrabarti A, Atassi R, Kardar AH, Osman MK, Husain I: Polyurethane internal ureteral stents in treatment of stone patients: morbidity related to indwelling times. *J. Urol.* 1991; 146: 1487-91.
[38] Kawahara T, Ito H, Terao H, Yoshida M, Matsuzaki J: Ureteral stent encrustation, incrustation, and coloring: morbidity related to indwelling times. *J. Endourol.* 2012; 26: 178-82.
[39] de Baere T, Denys A, Pappas P, Challier E, Roche A: Ureteral stents: exchange under fluoroscopic control as an effective alternative to cystoscopy. *Radiology.* 1994; 190: 887-9.
[40] Park SW, Cha IH, Hong SJ, Yi JG, Jeon HJ, Park JH, Park SJ: Fluoroscopy-guided transurethral removal and exchange of ureteral stents in female patients: technical notes. *J. Vasc. Interv. Radiol.* 2007; 18: 251-6.
[41] Kawahara T, Ito H, Terao H, Yamagishi T, Ogawa T, Uemura H, Kubota Y, Matsuzaki J: Ureteral stent retrieval using the crochet hook technique in females. *PloS. one.* 2012; 7: e29292.
[42] Kawahara T, Ito H, Terao H, Yamashita Y, Tanaka K, Ogawa T, Uemura H, Kubota Y, Matsuzaki J: Ureteral stent exchange under fluoroscopic guidance using the crochet hook technique in women. *Urol. Int.* 2012; 88: 322-5.

Chapter 7

Combination with PCNL: Ureteroscopy-Assisted Retrograde Nephrostomy (UARN)

Takashi Kawahara[*], M.D.[1,2,3], Hiroki Ito, M.D.[1,2],*
Hiroji Uemura, M.D., Ph.D.[2],
Yoshinobu Kubota, M.D., Ph.D.[2]
and Junichi Matsuzaki, M.D., Ph.D.[1]

[1]Department of Urology, Ohguchi Higashi General Hospital, Japan
[2]Department of Urology, Yokohama City University
Graduate School of Medicine, Japan
[3]Departments of Pathology and Urology,
Johns Hopkins University School of Medicine, Baltimore, Maryland, US

Abstract

Goodwin et al. first reported the ability to obtain percutaneous renal access in 1955. The technique for performing percutaneous nephrolithotomy (PCNL) was then developed, subsequently becoming

---

[*] Corresponding author: Takashi Kawahara, M.D. takashi_tk2001@yahoo.co.jp.

the standard procedure for treating large renal stones. Ultrasound-guided puncture of the renal collecting system with subsequent placement of a drainage tube under fluoroscopic guidance is currently the standard modality for performing percutaneous nephrostomy.

The development of rigid and flexible ureteroscopy (URS) has advanced the field of endoscopic ureteral surgery. We previously described a new technique for performing ureteroscopy (URS)-assisted retrograde nephrostomy (UARN) and experienced more than 100 cases. This procedure provides a higher stone-free rate, superior frequency of residual stones < 4 mm, lower incidence of complications and shorter operative time compared to previous percutaneous nephrostomy procedures. This chapter describes our experience with ureteroscopic assistance for PCNL.

Introduction

Retrograde nephrostomy was first developed by Lawson et al. in 1983, after which Hunter et al. reported 30 cases of retrograde nephrostomy in 1987 [1, 2].

Today, Lawson Retrograde Nephrostomy Wire Puncture Sets (COOK Urological, USA) can be easily obtained. This technique involves less radiation exposure and has a shorter procedural length than the previous percutaneous nephrostomy method.

For example, after the needle exits through the skin, no further steps are required in preparation for dilation [1, 3]. Retrograde nephrostomy using Lawson's procedure was first reported in the late 1980's by several authors [1-4]. However, since then, few studies of this procedure have been published due to the development of ultrasonography-assisted percutaneous nephrostomy [5].

With the arrival and development of flexible ureteroscopy (URS), both observation and manipulation in the renal pelvis can be easily achieved. We previously described a new technique for performing ureteroscopy (URS)-assisted retrograde nephrostomy (UARN).

This procedure involves less radiation exposure and a shorter operative time than the previous percutaneous nephrostomy method. Our technique represents an additional new option for performing percutaneous nephrolithotomy (PCNL) in patients with a nondilated intrarenal collecting system.

1. Procedure

Under general and epidural anesthesia, the patient is placed in a modified Valdivia position (Galdakao modified Valdivia position) [6-9]. Flexible URS (Flex-X^2, Tuttlingen, Karl Storz, Germany) insertion is carried out under an inserted ureteral access sheath in the ureter after ensuring that the semirigid URS (Uretero-renoscope, Karl Storz, Tuttlingen, Germany) does not encounter either ureteral stenosis or stones.

The UAS device includes a 12/14-Fr (inner/outer) 35-cm ureteral access sheath (UAS) (Flexor®, COOK Urological, IN, USA) or an 11/13-Fr 46-cm UAS (Navigator® 11 Fr 46 cm, Boston Scientific, MA, USA) placed in the ureter.

We carefully observe the target calculi and select the appropriate renal calyx to puncture. Thereafter, a Lawson retrograde nephrostomy puncture wire (Lawson Retrograde Nephrostomy Wire Puncture Set, COOK Urological, IN, USA) is carefully placed into the flexible URS [2]. The URS approaches the desired renal calyx a second time, and the route from the renal calyx to the exit site on the skin is then confirmed under fluoroscopy.

In order to avoid injury to the spleen, liver, intestines or pleural cavity, a puncture is then performed under ultrasonography after rechecking the preoperative CT scan.

The puncture wire is easily passed through the muscle and "tents" the skin at the posterior axial line. The skin is then incised, and the needle is delivered. Next, the dilator is placed using the puncture wire, which is advanced through the skin, subcutaneous fat, abdominal wall musculature and perinephric fat until it reaches the renal parenchyma. Subsequently, a 22-G and 18-G needle dilator is placed over the puncture wire, which is advanced through the skin, subcutaneous fat, abdominal wall musculature and perinephric fat until it reaches the renal parenchyma.

The catheter is dilated up to 12 Fr, and a safety guidewire is placed through the UAS. A 24-Fr percutaneous nephro-access sheath (X-Force®N30 Nephrostomy Balloon Dilation Catheter, BARD, USA) is passed over the balloon into the calyx under ureteroscopic and fluoroscopic guidance, after which the balloon is removed. Calculus fragmentation is performed using the Swiss LithoClast® pneumatic lithotripter (EMS, Nyon, Switzerland) through a rigid nephroscope (percutaneous nephroscope, Karl Storz, Tuttlingen, Germany).

2. UARN for PCNL

Goodwin et al. first reported the ability to obtain percutaneous renal access in 1955 [10]. The technique of percutaneous nephrolithotomy (PCNL) was then developed, subsequently becoming the standard procedure for treating large renal stones. Ultrasound-guided puncture of the renal collecting system with subsequent placement of a drainage tube under fluoroscopic guidance is currently the standard modality for performing percutaneous nephrostomy.

Even when percutaneous access is successfully obtained in a patient with a non-dilated collecting system using needle puncture, the tract is often not situated in the most desirable location for stone extraction [2]. Retrograde nephrostomy was first developed by Lawson et al. in 1983, after which Hunter et al. reported 30 cases of retrograde nephrostomy in 1985 [1, 2]. In this procedure, after the needle has exited through the skin, no further steps are required in preparation for dilation. We investigated the impact of UARN during PCNL on the stone-free rate, frequency of residual stones measuring < 4 mm, operative time, reoperative risk and complications in patients with large renal stones (stone burden > 2.0 cm) [11].

Between April 2009 and September 2011, a total of 50 patients underwent PCNL for large renal stones (stone burden > 2 cm). Among these patients, we performed UARN in the Galdakao-modified Valdivia position in 27 patients (UARN PCNL group) and ultrasonography (US)-assisted nephrostomy in the prone position in 23 patients (prone PCNL group). This study was approved by the Institutional Review Board of Ohguchi Higashi General Hospital, and informed consent was obtained from all participants. Prone PCNL was performed between April 2009 and March 2011, and UARN PCNL was performed between August 2010 and September 2011. Between August 2010 and March 2011, which was a period of transition from prone PCNL to UARN PCNL, prone PCNL was performed in five cases and UARN PCNL was performed in four cases. The exclusion criteria included a previous history of nephrostomy, shockwave lithotomy (SWL), URS or PCNL.

Fifty patients included in this study (27 in the UARN PCNL group and 23 in the prone PCNL group) had a renal stone burden of > 2.0 cm. All stone locations were renal. The median stone burden was 57 mm (mean: 59.1 ± 28.1 mm) in the UARN PCNL group and 51 mm (mean: 57.6 ± 20.7 mm) in the prone PCNL group. The median maximum stone size was 32 mm (mean: 32.7 ± 13.5 mm) in the UARN PCNL group and 37 mm (mean: 38.2 ± 13.2 mm) in the prone PCNL group. UARN PCNL significantly improved the stone-free rate and frequency of residual stones < 4 mm ($P = 0.027$ and $P = 0.015$, respectively). The median operative time was significantly shorter in the UARN PCNL group, at 160 minutes (mean: 187.1 ± 77.4 min) compared to 299 minutes (mean: 297.5 ± 100.4 min) in the prone PCNL group. Completion of the initial treatment was achieved in 17 of the 22 patients (62.9%) in the UARN PCNL group and eight of the 23 patients (34.8%) in the prone PCNL group. The UARN PCNL group therefore exhibited a higher rate of completion during the initial treatment, although the difference was not significant ($P = 0.048$). Postoperative complications included a high-grade fever that persisted for three days in two patients (7.4%) in the UARN PCNL group and six patients (26.1%) in the prone PCNL group. None of the UARN PCNL patients had a Clavien score of ≥ 3.

In the present study, we continuously and easily visualized the motion of the ureteroscope under ultrasonography and were able to detect the tent sign without changing the patient's position. Using our procedure, after the needle has exited through the skin, no further steps are required in preparation for dilation. In addition, UARN provides continuous visualization from puncture to PCNL, including needle, catheter and balloon dilation and insertion of the nephron-access sheath. This procedure provides a higher stone-free rate, a superior frequency of residual stones < 4 mm, a lower incidence of complications and a shorter operative time than previous percutaneous nephrostomy procedures.

3. Procedures for Complicated Cases

3.1. Obese Patients

Although no disadvantages of PCNL have so far been reported in obese patients, in general, obesity is associated with increased surgical morbidity and mortality [12]. PCNL is usually performed with the patient in the prone position [12]. In morbidly obese patients, this position can exacerbate respiratory compromise and impede venous return [13]. In response to these problems, the use of PCNL in the supine position was recently reported and become well established [6, 14]. UARN is performed continuously under visualization with URS and fluoroscopy, which allows for adequate puncture and the ability to easily change directions without extracting the puncture wire.

Therefore, performing nephrostomy in an ideal position can be achieved. In addition, this procedure does not require position changes from the lithotomy position to the prone position and vice versa [15].

3.2. Patients Treated with Anatrophic Nephrolithotomy

Until the development of endoscopic devices and endoscopic techniques, open surgical anatrophic nephrolithotomy (ANL) was the standard treatment for large renal calculi. ANL performed with formal plastic calyrhaphy and/or calycoplasty was first described by Smith and Boyce in 1968 [16]. Since then, Matlaga and Assimos reported a stone-free rate of 100% using open stone surgery to treat staghorn renal stones [17]. Following advances in laparoscopic techniques, the use of laparoscopic ANL was recently reported [18-20]. Due to the invasiveness of ANL and the risk of postoperative adhesion, performing repeated ANL is difficult in patients with recurrent renal stones. In our institute, we perform PCNL using the UARN technique in patients with a history of ANL. Due to the potential for intraoperative separation and postoperative adhesion following ANL, the renal position is relocated to the dorsal side and puncture is performed from the middle calyx on the dorsal side. A potential disadvantage of this procedure is the danger of exiting the kidney in the ventral direction, with possible injury to the intestines [3]. We performed the puncture under ultrasonographic and fluoroscopic guidance in order to avoid injury to the surrounding organs. UARN is also a safe and effective approach in patients with a history of ANL [21].

3.3. Patients with a Horseshoe Kidney

Horseshoe kidney is the most common renal fusion anomaly, with a prevalence of 0.25% of the population [22]. Ureteroscopy (URS) has been successfully performed in some cases, although due to the altered anatomical relationships observed in such patients, the use of ureteroscopic approaches is often quite challenging and not universally recommended [23, 24]. In order to reach to the lower calix, nephrostomy is usually performed in the upper calix. In patients with a horseshoe kidney, Raj G.V. et al. and Al-Otabi et al. reported that 15 of 24 patients (64%) and nine of 12 patients (75%) required nephrostomy in the upper calix, respectively [22, 25]. The presence of an upper pole nephrostomy tract allows for enhanced intrarenal access to the upper pole calix, renal pelvis, lower pole calix, ureteropelvic junction and proximal ureter [22]. The disadvantage of performing nephrostomy in the upper calix is that the procedure sometimes requires a longer distance from the skin to the lower calix, such that the nephroscope is unable to reach to the target stone [22, 26]. In addition, Raj G.V. et al. reported a rate of pneumothorax complications of 6% among patients treated with nephrostomy in the upper calix [22]. Therefore, performing an accurate puncture in the upper calix is required. We speculate that UARN is effective for obtaining an accurate puncture site from the desired calix to the skin. Therefore, this technique is thus considered to positively contribute to the performance of an ideal nephrostomy procedure in the upper calix during PCNL in patients with a horseshoe kidney [27].

3.4. Patients with Complete Staghorn Stones

Complete staghorn calculi are usually managed with percutaneous nephrolithotomy; however, performing dilating nephrostomy and inserting the nephron-access sheath are sometimes very difficult in patients without hydronephrosis. Staghorn calculi are branched stones that occupy a large portion of the collecting system. A complete staghorn calculus refers to a stone that occupies virtually the entire collecting system. In our experience with one case, the calculus fully occupied all renal calices. Therefore, we speculate that placing the guidewire in the ureter before dilation is very difficult, even when percutaneous nephrostomy using ultrasonography or fluoroscopically is successful. Therefore, UARN may be a new option for performing PCNL in patients with complete staghorn stones.

3.5. Patients with an Incomplete Double Ureter

The incidence of a double renal pelvis and ureter ranges from 0.5% to 3.0% in humans [28, 29]. The anomalies of duplication of the ureter and pelvis are classified as complete or incomplete [28, 29]. Incomplete duplication is three times more common than complete duplication. In incomplete duplication, wherein the pelvis and two ureters join together and enter the bladder via one common orifice, both forms of duplication may be unilateral or bilateral. Patients with duplication of the ureter exhibit an increased risk of stone formation [30]. Performing PCNL in patients with an abnormal kidney is sometimes difficult, in particular among those without hydronephrosis. The use of UARN facilitates continuous visualization from puncture to insertion of the nephron-access sheath in patients treated with URS. In such cases, URS contributes to the ability to visualize the detailed anatomy surrounding the punctured calyx and target stone. Therefore, UARN is considered to be a potentially useful new option for performing PCNL in patients with ureteral duplication [31].

3.6. Patients with an Ileal Conduit

The use of an appliance for diversion, such as an ileal conduit or cutaneous ureterostomy, is primarily considered in patients undergoing radical cystectomy who are not candidates for continent diversion procedures [32]. However, a significant number of patients experience complications associated with ileal conduit diversion. In addition, ureteral calculi develop in 10.7% of patients at a later stage, while ureteroileal obstruction is observed in 4% to 7.9% of cases [33, 34]. We perform PCNL using UARN in patients with an ileal conduit. An occlusion catheter is usually used in those with a nondilated renal collecting system. However, inserting an occlusion catheter is difficult in patients with a history of urinary diversion. Therefore, flexible cystoscopy or URS is used to approach the ureter, and UARN is ideal for treating patients without a dilated renal collecting system.

Conclusion

Due to the development of endoscopic and surrounding devices, the ureteroscopic management of urolithiasis is currently safe and effective. UARN, in combination with ureteroscopy, is a potential new option for treating complicated cases of renal stones.

References

[1] Hunter PT, Finlayson B, Drylie DM, Leal J, Hawkins IF. Retrograde nephrostomy and percutaneous calculus removal in 30 patients. *J. Urol.* 1985; 133: 369-74.

[2] Lawson RK, Murphy JB, Taylor AJ, Jacobs SC. Retrograde method for percutaneous access to kidney. *Urology.* 1983; 22: 580-2.
[3] Hawkins IF, Jr., Hunter P, Leal G, Nanni G, Hawkins M, Finlayson B, Senior D. Retrograde nephrostomy for stone removal: combined cystoscopic/percutaneous technique. *Am. J. Roentgenol.* 1984; 143: 299-304.
[4] Spirnak JP, Resnick MI. Retrograde percutaneous stone removal using modified Lawson technique. *Urology.* 1987; 30: 551-3.
[5] Agarwal M, Agrawal MS, Jaiswal A, Kumar D, Yadav H, Lavania P. Safety and efficacy of ultrasonography as an adjunct to fluoroscopy for renal access in percutaneous nephrolithotomy (PCNL). *BJU. Int.* 2011; 108: 1346-9.
[6] Valdivia Uria JG, Lachares Santamaria E, Villarroya Rodriguez S, Taberner Llop J, Abril Baquero G, Aranda Lassa JM. Percutaneous nephrolithectomy: simplified technic (preliminary report). *Arch. Esp. Urol.* 1987; 40: 177-80.
[7] Valdivia Uria JG, Valle Gerhold J, Lopez Lopez JA, Villarroya Rodriguez S, Ambroj Navarro C, Ramirez Fabian M, Rodriguez Bazalo JM, Sanchez Elipe MA. Technique and complications of percutaneous nephroscopy: experience with 557 patients in the supine position. *J. Urol.* 1998; 160: 1975-8.
[8] Scoffone CM, Cracco CM, Cossu M, Grande S, Poggio M, Scarpa RM. Endoscopic combined intrarenal surgery in Galdakao-modified supine Valdivia position: a new standard for percutaneous nephrolithotomy? *Eur. Urol.* 2008; 54: 1393-403.
[9] Daels F, Gonzalez MS, Freire FG, Jurado A, Damia O. Percutaneous lithotripsy in Valdivia-Galdakao decubitus position: our experience. *J. Endourol.* 2009; 23: 1615-20.
[10] Goodwin WE, Casey WC, Woolf W: Percutaneous trocar (needle) nephrostomy in hydronephrosis. *J. Am. Med. Assoc.* 1955; 157: 891-4.
[11] Kawahara T, Ito H, Terao H, Kato Y, Uemura H, Kubota Y, Matsuzaki J. Effectiveness of ureteroscopy-assisted retrograde nephrostomy (UARN) for percutaneous nephrolithotomy (PCNL). *PloS. one.* 2012; 7: e52149.
[12] El-Assmy AM, Shokeir AA, El-Nahas AR, Shoma AM, Eraky I, El-Kenawy MR, El-Kappany HA. Outcome of percutaneous nephrolithotomy: effect of body mass index. *Eur. Urol.* 2007; 52: 199-204.

[13] Gofrit ON, Shapiro A, Donchin Y, Bloom AI, Shenfeld OZ, Landau EH, Pode D. Lateral decubitus position for percutaneous nephrolithotripsy in the morbidly obese or kyphotic patient. *J. Endourol.* 2002; 16: 383-6.
[14] Valdivia JG, Scarpa RM, Duvdevani M, Gross AJ, Nadler RB, Nutahara K, de la Rosette, On Behalf Of The Croes Pcnl Study Group JJ. Supine Versus Prone Position During Percutaneous Nephrolithotomy: A Report from the Clinical Research Office of the Endourological Society Percutaneous Nephrolithotomy Global Study. *J. Endourol.* 2011; 25: 1619-25.
[15] Kawahara T, Matsuzaki J, Kubota Y. Ureteroscopy-assisted retrograde nephrostomy for an obese patient. *Indian. J. Urol.* 2012; 28: 439-41.
[16] Smith MJ, Boyce WH. Anatrophic nephrotomy and plastic calyrhaphy. *J. Urol.* 1968; 99: 521-7.
[17] Matlaga BR, Assimos DG. Changing indications of open stone surgery. *Urology.* 2002; 59: 490-3.
[18] Melissourgos ND, Davilas EN, Fragoulis A, Kiminas E, Farmakis A. Modified anatrophic nephrolithotomy for complete staghorn calculus disease -- does it still have a place? *Scand. J. Urol. Nephrol.* 2002; 36: 426-30.
[19] Zhou L, Xuan Q, Wu B, Xiao J, Dong X, Huang T, Chen H, Zhu Y, Wu K. Retroperitoneal laparoscopic anatrophic nephrolithotomy for large staghorn calculi. *Int. J. Urol.* 2011; 18: 126-9.
[20] Simforoosh N, Aminsharifi A, Tabibi A, Noor-Alizadeh A, Zand S, Radfar MH, Javaherforooshzadeh A. Laparoscopic anatrophic nephrolithotomy for managing large staghorn calculi. *BJU. Int.* 2008; 101: 1293-6.
[21] Kawahara T, Ito H, Terao H, Kato Y, Ogawa T, Uemura H, Kubota Y, Matsuzaki J. Ureteroscopy-Assisted Retrograde Nephrostomy (UARN) after Anatrophic Nephrolithotomy. *Case. Rep. Med.* 2012; 2012: 164963.
[22] Raj GV, Auge BK, Weizer AZ, Denstedt JD, Watterson JD, Beiko DT, Assimos DG, Preminger GM. Percutaneous management of calculi within horseshoe kidneys. *J. Urol.* 2003; 170: 48-51.
[23] Esuvaranathan K, Tan EC, Tung KH, Foo KT. Stones in horseshoe kidneys: results of treatment by extracorporeal shock wave lithotripsy and endourology. *J. Urol.* 1991; 146: 1213-5.
[24] Andreoni C, Portis AJ, Clayman RV. Retrograde renal pelvic access sheath to facilitate flexible ureteroscopic lithotripsy for the treatment of urolithiasis in a horseshoe kidney. *J. Urol.* 2000; 164: 1290-1.

[25] Al-Otaibi K, Hosking DH. Percutaneous stone removal in horseshoe kidneys. *J. Urol.* 1999; 162: 674-7.
[26] El Ghoneimy MN, Kodera AS, Emran AM, Orban TZ, Shaban AM, El Gammal MM. Percutaneous nephrolithotomy in horseshoe kidneys: is rigid nephroscopy sufficient tool for complete clearance? A case series study. *BMC. Urol.* 2009; 9: 17.
[27] Kawahara T, Ito H, Terao H, Tanaka K, Ogawa T, Uemura H, Kubota Y, Matsuzaki J. Ureteroscopy-assisted retrograde nephrostomy for lower calyx calculi in horseshoe kidney: two case reports. *J. Med. Case. Rep.* 2012; 6: 194.
[28] Wakeley CP. A Case of Duplication of the Ureters. *J. Anat. Physiol.* 1915; 49: 148-54.
[29] Inamoto K, Tanaka S, Takemura K, Ikoma F. Duplication of the renal pelvis and ureter: associated anomalies and pathological conditions. *Radiat. Med.* 1983; 1: 55-64.
[30] Ahmed S, Pope R. Uncrossed complete ureteral duplication with upper system reflux. *J. Urol.* 1986; 135: 128-9.
[31] Kawahara T, Ito H, Terao H, Kato Y, Ogawa T, Uemura H, Kubota Y, Matsuzaki J. Ureteroscopy-assisted retrograde nephrostomy (UARN) for an incomplete double ureter. *Urologic. Res.* 2012; 40: 781-2.
[32] Rodriguez AR, Lockhart A, King J, Wiegand L, Carrion R, Ordorica R, Lockhart J. Cutaneous ureterostomy technique for adults and effects of ureteral stenting: an alternative to the ileal conduit. *J. Urol.* 2011; 186: 1939-43.
[33] Schmidt JD, Hawtrey CE, Flocks RH, Culp DA. Complications, results and problems of ileal conduit diversions. *J. Urol.* 1973; 109: 210-6.
[34] Vandenbroucke F, Van Poppel H, Vandeursen H, Oyen R, Baert L. Surgical versus endoscopic treatment of non-malignant uretero-ileal anastomotic strictures. *Br. J. Urol.* 1993; 71: 408-12.

PART IV. EVALUATIONS

Chapter 8

Pre- and Post-Operative Evaluations

Hiroki Ito[*], M.D.[1,2], Takashi Kawahara, M.D.[1,2,3],
Masahiro Yao, M.D., Ph.D.[2],
Yoshinobu Kubota, M.D., Ph.D.[2]
and Junichi Matsuzaki, M.D., Ph.D.[1]*

[1]Department of Urology, Ohguchi East General Hospital
[2]Department of Urology, Yokohama City University
Graduate School of Medicine
[3]Departments of Pathology and Urology,
Johns Hopkins University School of Medicine, Baltimore, Maryland, US

Abstract

Recently, the therapeutic potential of surgery for the treatment of urinary stones has improved in association with the development of several surgical devices. Accordingly, the assessment of a patient's stone status plays an important role in the management of urinary stones, particularly before surgical intervention. Among some modalities for imaging, non-contrast computed tomography (NCCT) showed high

---

[*] Corresponding author: Hiroki Ito, M.D. pug_daikichi@yahoo.co.jp.

sensitivity and specificity, therefore is most frequently used in the initial diagnosis of urinary stones as well as assessments before and after surgical intervention. Several parameters obtained on preoperative imaging provide beneficial information for predicting the surgical outcome. Previous reports have indicated that the stone burden, stone location or attenuation coefficients on NCCT were the predictor of the outcome of surgical intervention. In this chapter, we reviewed the role and utility of imaging in the treatment of urinary stones, particularly before and after surgery.

Introduction

Patients with urinary calculi often undergo repeated imaging studies in order to determine the diagnosis. Furthermore, patients with urinary stones are at high risk of recurrence (with a recurrence rate approaching 50% [1]); therefore, providing follow-up with repeated imaging is necessary [2, 3]. Recently, the therapeutic potential of surgery for the treatment of urinary stones has improved in association with the development of several surgical devices. Accordingly, it is important to evaluate the stone status using imaging modalities before, during and after treatment, including ureteroscopy (URS) [4]. In this chapter, we describe the role of imaging in the treatment of urinary stones, particularly before and after URS.

1. Imaging Modalities for Evaluating Urinary Stones

1.1. Non-contrast computed tomography (NCCT)

The best imaging modality for confirming the diagnosis of a urinary stone in patients with acute flank pain is NCCT, which has been reported to be the most sensitive and specific modality for detecting the size and location of urinary stones [5-8]. The advantages of CT in detecting urinary stones have been clearly established, including a high contrast resolution allowing for the detection of almost all stones, except for certain complications of triple combination therapy in HIV-seropositive patients, extensive cover facilitating the identification of differential diagnoses, rapidity and enhanced efficacy and finally the absence of risk related to the injection of iodinated contrast agents.

Therefore, NCCT is frequently used in the initial diagnosis of urinary stones as well as assessments before surgical intervention [4, 9, 10] and the follow-up of known urinary stones before and after treatment.

1.2. Low-dose NCCT

The use of low-dose CT (< 4 mSv) is preferred in patients with a BMI of 30 kg/m2 or less, as this modification of standard CT imaging limits the potential long-term side effects of ionizing radiation while maintaining a sensitivity and specificity of 90% or greater [11-13]. However, low-dose CT is not recommended in those with a BMI greater than 30 kg/m2 due to the lower sensitivity and specificity for detecting urinary stones [11]. Females in the second and third trimesters are candidates for low-dose CT if ultrasonography (US) is not diagnostic [14].

1.3. Kidney-Ureter-Bladder (KUB) Films

Follow-up KUB is performed in patients who are candidates for observation and those in whom a stone was identified on the initial KUB examination, as this modality provides an indication of stone progression. The use of follow-up KUB should also be considered in subjects in whom no stones were observed on the initial KUB study because the stone(s) were positioned in the sacroiliac area, thus limiting visualization. Oblique films may also be obtained in such cases, at either the time of the original CT scan or follow-up, as these images may further facilitate stone visualization. Certain parameters and findings should be assessed on CT imaging in order to facilitate subsequent management decisions. Alternative imaging modalities are considered in specific patient groups. The combination of US and KUB is a viable option in patients with a known stone who have previously exhibited radiopaque stones [15, 16].

1.4. Ultrasonography (US)

Renal US, despite its lower sensitivity, is the preferred initial imaging modality for children and pregnant females with suspected colic pain due to radiation concerns [17-20]. Low-dose CT is an alternative if renal US is not diagnostic in children in whom a ureteral stone is suspected [21, 22]. If the diagnosis is not established with this modality during the first trimester, magnetic resonance imaging without contrast [23] or URS [24] should be considered as a second-line imaging examination, as the fetus is most susceptible to potential radiation-induced injury in the first trimester.

1.5. Intravenous Urography (IVU)

In cases in which hydronephrosis is present with a known ureteral calculus, IVU is primarily used to assess the renal obstruction/function [2]. However, IVU has been gradually replaced in recent years as the "gold standard" method for assessing the renal parenchyma and urinary tract by US and NCCT. The current place of IVU in patients with renal colic is therefore to establish a definitive diagnosis and guide urgent procedures when other modalities are unavailable. The essential indication remains detailed visualization of the urinary tract, detailed visualization of the entire urinary tract or even the gross assessment of the renal function in patients with multiple injuries that cannot be investigated using CT and in whom the surgeon rightly hesitates before opening the retroperitoneum [25].

2. Pre-Operative Imaging Predictors of the Outcome of URS

The assessment of a patient's stone status plays an important role in the management of urinary stones, particularly before surgical intervention. Several parameters obtained on preoperative imaging provide beneficial information for predicting the surgical outcome. In this section, we review the utility of preoperative imaging indicators.

2.1. Stone Burden

Many previous reports have indicated that the stone burden is the best predictor of the outcome of surgical intervention. Several stone parameters reflecting the stone burden, including the cumulative maximum diameter, surface area and volume, have been assessed in studies of URS [26, 27]. Based on area under the receiver operating curve (AUROC) analyses, three parameters of the stone burden have been found to have a high sensitivity and specificity (Figure 1) [4, 10, 28].

2.2. Stone Location

The stone location is another primary contributor to the success of URS. Many reports have demonstrated that the presence of proximal ureteral stones [29] and lower pole calculi of renal stones [4] is a significant predictor of failure of URS due to the movement of the stones and restrictions in the treatable angle obtained with URS. Recently, however, Takazawa R. et al. showed that, with advances in URS, the stone location no longer has a strong influence on the outcome of URS [30].

2.3. Hydronephrosis

As a standard, current guidelines [3] recommend that patients "should be followed with periodic imaging studies to monitor the stone position and assess for hydronephrosis." A panel sought to validate the reliability of hydronephrosis as a proxy for the degree of obstruction in patients with suspected ureteral calculi. The majority of patients with ureteral stones have some degree of hydronephrosis. The presence and/or degree of hydronephrosis have been shown to influence the results of shock wave lithotripsy of ureteral stones, although these findings have less impact on ureteroscopic removal [29, 31].

2.4. Attenuation Coefficients on NCCT

Our previous study showed that both the maximum and average attenuation coefficients on NCCT are significantly related to the fragmentation efficiency (Figure 2) [32]. The fragmentation efficiency represents the degree of stone fragility during URS using holmium laser lithotripsy and is strongly associated with the operative time required to break the stones into the desired size of fragments. In addition, our previous study also showed that, in patients with stone a burden of <20.0 mm in diameter, both the maximum and average attenuation coefficients are significantly predictive of the operative time [32].

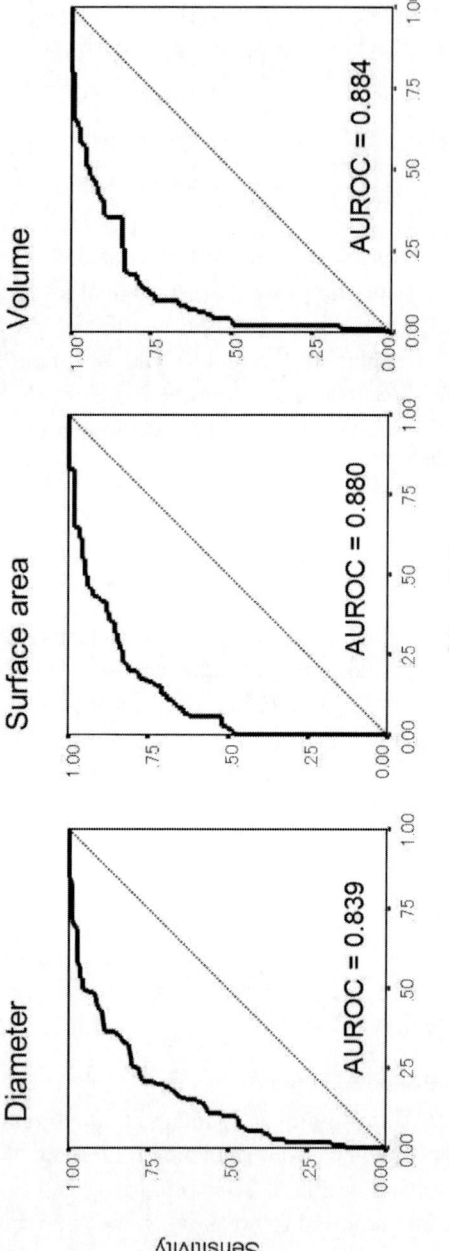

Figure 1. Receiver operating characteristics (ROC) curves of the stone-free (SF) status on postoperative day (POD) 1 for the cumulative stone diameter (CSD), stone surface area (SA) and stone volume (N=238) (cited from reference [4] and modified).

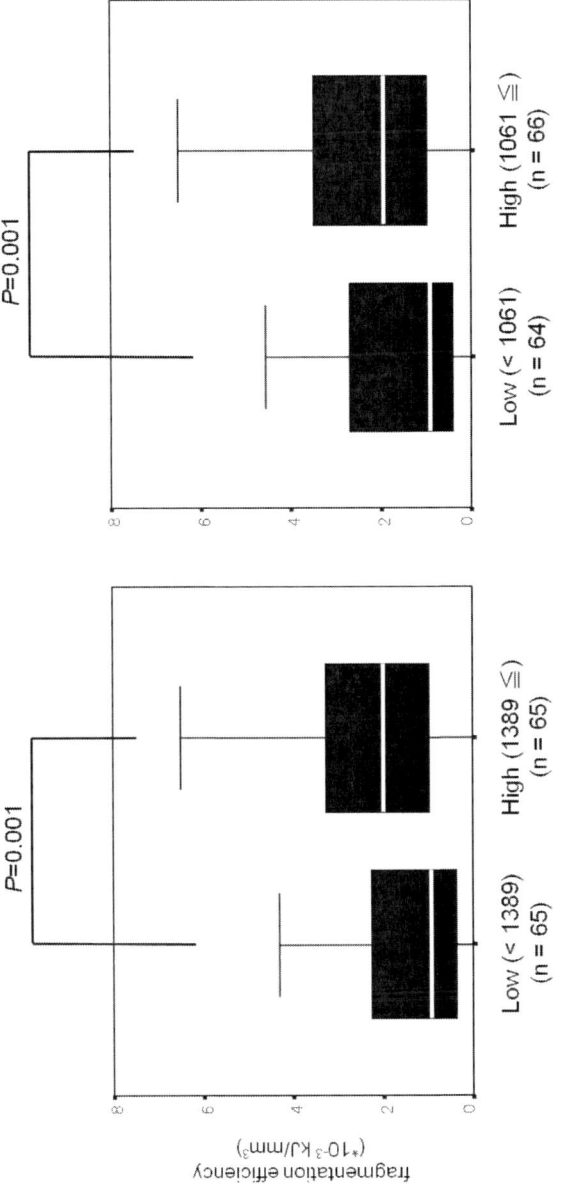

Figure 2. Boxplot of the fragmentation efficiency comparing low and high maximum and average attenuation coefficients (cited from reference [32] and modified).

However, neither the maximum nor average attenuation coefficient have been found to be correlated in patients with a stone burden of >20.0 mm in diameter. This finding suggests that the operative time can be directly predicted based on pretreatment measurements of the attenuation coefficient on NCCT in patients with a lower stone burden, particularly that involving a burden of <20.0 mm in diameter.

Previous studies have reported the average attenuation coefficient cutoff point predicting ESWL failure to be set from 750 to 1,000 HU, which varies little from study to study [33-35]. In our previous study, we set the overall median value of each attenuation coefficient (maximum: 1,389 HU, average: 1,061 HU) as the cutoff point for each group and found these cutoff points to be appropriate due to their effectiveness as predictors of the surgical outcome (Figure 2) [32]. These findings suggest that the cutoff points for URS are similar to those for ESWL.

3. Post-URS Follow-Up Imaging

Following definitive surgical intervention for urinary stones, follow-up imaging is provided in order to assure complete stone removal and/or the absence of obstruction. Ureteral instrumentation and particularly stone fragmentation warrant postoperative imaging to document the clearance of the stone fragments, resolution of hydronephrosis and/or development of unanticipated obstruction, such as that due to ureteral stricture. Although the incidence of ureteral stricture after URS is low, its occurrence is not entirely predictable [3, 36]. In most reports, ureteral stricture has been shown to be likely the result of adjunctive instrumentation or stone impaction. Although the need for imaging studies to confirm stone fragment clearance after URS with lithotripsy is widely accepted, the need for follow-up studies in asymptomatic patients to assess for obstruction is a subject of debate. Moreover, the timing of follow-up imaging studies and the need for secondary intervention is left to the discretion of the treating physician.

3.1. Imaging in Postoperatively Asymptomatic Patients

Several previous studies have indicated that the incidence of postoperative obstruction in asymptomatic patients is decidedly low [36-39]. In patients who have undergone URS with stone fragmentation and are currently asymptomatic, follow-up imaging with US and KUB can be used to document the presence of residual fragments and/or hydronephrosis. In the absence of hydronephrosis and residual fragments, no further imaging is indicated. However, in patients with radiopaque stones, if residual fragments and/or hydronephrosis are documented, further observation or intervention should be pursued at the discretion of the practitioner [2].

In patients with non-opaque stones, the presence of hydronephrosis on a US should prompt a further evaluation with low-dose NCCT in order to identify obstructive residual fragments. However, silent obstruction remains a potentially significant complication after stone management [36].

Relying on the patient's report of postoperative pain to determine the need for postoperative imaging places the patient at risk for progressive renal failure due to unrecognized obstruction. Therefore, a previous report recommended performing imaging of the collecting system using IVU, NCCT and/or US within three months after routine ureteroscopic stone treatment in order to prevent the potential complications of unrecognized ureteral obstruction [2].

3.2. Imaging in Postoperatively Symptomatic Patients

Obstruction with or without associated symptoms after URS is generally caused by the accumulation of obstructive stone fragments or ureteral stricture. With the low incidence of stricture, the presence of obstructive fragments is likely to be the more common etiology overall and may be detectable with repeated imaging (KUB, NCCT or low-dose NCCT), thereby providing a means of identifying patients requiring further functional imaging and/or secondary treatment [2].

Conclusion

We reviewed the role and utility of imaging in the treatment of urinary stones, particularly before and after URS.

References

[1] Sierakowski R, Finlayson B, Landes RR, Finlayson CD, Sierakowski N. The frequency of urolithiasis in hospital discharge diagnoses in the United States. *Invest. Urol.* 1978; 15: 438-41.

[2] Fulgham PF, Assimos DG, Pearle MS, Preminger GM. Clinical effectiveness protocols for imaging in the management of ureteral calculous disease: AUA technology assessment. *J. Urol.* 2013; 189: 1203-13.

[3] Preminger GM, Tiselius HG, Assimos DG, Alken P, Buck C, Gallucci M, et al. 2007 guideline for the management of ureteral calculi. *J. Urol.* 2007; 178: 2418-34.

[4] Ito H, Kawahara T, Terao H, Ogawa T, Yao M, Kubota Y, et al. The most reliable preoperative assessment of renal stone burden as a predictor of stone-free status after flexible ureteroscopy with holmium laser lithotripsy: a single-center experience. *Urology.* 2012; 80: 524-8.

[5] Narepalem N, Sundaram CP, Boridy IC, Yan Y, Heiken JP, Clayman RV. Comparison of helical computerized tomography and plain radiography for estimating urinary stone size. *J. Urol.* 2002; 167: 1235-8.

[6] Parsons JK, Lancini V, Shetye K, Regan F, Potter SR, Jarrett TW. Urinary stone size: comparison of abdominal plain radiography and noncontrast CT measurements. *J. Endourol.* 2003; 17: 725-8.

[7] Dundee P, Bouchier-Hayes D, Haxhimolla H, Dowling R, Costello A. Renal tract calculi: comparison of stone size on plain radiography and noncontrast spiral CT scan. *J. Endourol.* 2006; 20: 1005-9.

[8] Vieweg J, Teh C, Freed K, Leder RA, Smith RH, Nelson RH, et al. Unenhanced helical computerized tomography for the evaluation of patients with acute flank pain. *J. Urol.* 1998; 160: 679-84.

[9] Hyams ES, Korley FK, Pham JC, Matlaga BR. Trends in imaging use during the emergency department evaluation of flank pain. *J. Urol.* 2011; 186: 2270-4.

[10] Ito H, Kawahara T, Terao H, Ogawa T, Yao M, Kubota Y, et al. Utility and limitation of cumulative stone diameter in predicting urinary stone burden at flexible ureteroscopy with holmium laser lithotripsy: a single-center experience. *PloS one.* 2013; 8: e65060.

[11] Hamm M, Knopfle E, Wartenberg S, Wawroschek F, Weckermann D, Harzmann R. Low dose unenhanced helical computerized tomography for the evaluation of acute flank pain. *J. Urol.* 2002; 167: 1687-91.
[12] Heneghan JP, McGuire KA, Leder RA, DeLong DM, Yoshizumi T, Nelson RC. Helical CT for nephrolithiasis and ureterolithiasis: comparison of conventional and reduced radiation-dose techniques. *Radiology.* 2003; 229: 575-80.
[13] Kim BS, Hwang IK, Choi YW, Namkung S, Kim HC, Hwang WC, et al. Low-dose and standard-dose unenhanced helical computed tomography for the assessment of acute renal colic: prospective comparative study. *Acta Radiol.* 2005; 46: 756-63.
[14] White WM, Zite NB, Gash J, Waters WB, Thompson W, Klein FA. Low-dose computed tomography for the evaluation of flank pain in the pregnant population. *J. Endourol.* 2007; 21: 1255-60.
[15] Shokeir AA, El-Diasty T, Eassa W, Mosbah A, El-Ghar MA, Mansour O, et al. Diagnosis of ureteral obstruction in patients with compromised renal function: the role of noninvasive imaging modalities. *J. Urology.* 2004; 171: 2303-6.
[16] Ripolles T, Agramunt M, Errando J, Martinez MJ, Coronel B, Morales M. Suspected ureteral colic: plain film and sonography vs unenhanced helical CT. A prospective study in 66 patients. *Eur. Radiol.* 2004; 14: 129-36.
[17] Elgamasy A, Elsherif A. Use of Doppler ultrasonography and rigid ureteroscopy for managing symptomatic ureteric stones during pregnancy. *BJU international.* 2010; 106: 262-6.
[18] Elwagdy S, Ghoneim S, Moussa S, Ewis I. Three-dimensional ultrasound (3D US) methods in the evaluation of calcular and non-calcular ureteric obstructive uropathy. *World J. Urol.* 2008; 26: 263-74.
[19] Pepe F, Pepe P. Color Doppler ultrasound (CDU) in the diagnosis of obstructive hydronephrosis in pregnant women. *Arch. Gynecol. Obst.* 2013; 288: 489-93.
[20] Shokeir AA, Mahran MR, Abdulmaaboud M. Renal colic in pregnant women: role of renal resistive index. *Urology.* 2000; 55: 344-7.
[21] Passerotti C, Chow JS, Silva A, Schoettler CL, Rosoklija I, Perez-Rossello J, et al. Ultrasound versus computerized tomography for evaluating urolithiasis. *J. Urol.* 2009; 182(4 Suppl): 1829-34.
[22] Palmer JS, Donaher ER, O'Riordan MA, Dell KM. Diagnosis of pediatric urolithiasis: role of ultrasound and computerized tomography. *J. Urol.* 2005; 174: 1413-6.

[23] Masselli G, Derme M, Laghi F, Polettini E, Brunelli R, Framarino ML, et al. Imaging of stone disease in pregnancy. *Abd. Imag.* 2013; 38: 1409-14.
[24] Isen K, Hatipoglu NK, Dedeoglu S, Atilgan I, Caca FN, Hatipoglu N. Experience with the diagnosis and management of symptomatic ureteric stones during pregnancy. *Urology.* 2012; 79: 508-12.
[25] Laissy JP, Abecidan E, Karila-Cohen P, Ravery V, Schouman-Claeys E. IVU: a test of the past without future? *Progres en urologie.* 2001; 11: 552-61.
[26] Hyams ES, Bruhn A, Lipkin M, Shah O. Heterogeneity in the reporting of disease characteristics and treatment outcomes in studies evaluating treatments for nephrolithiasis. *J. Endourol.* 2010; 24: 1411-4.
[27] Kawahara T, Ito H, Terao H, Ogawa T, Uemura H, Kubota Y, et al. Stone area and volume are correlated with operative time for cystolithotripsy for bladder calculi using a holmium: yttrium garnet laser. *Scand. J. Urol. Nephrol.* 2012; 46: 298-303..
[28] Ito H, Kawahara T, Terao H, Ogawa T, Yao M, Kubota Y, et al. Evaluation of preoperative measurement of stone surface area as a predictor of stone-free status after combined ureteroscopy with holmium laser lithotripsy: a single-center experience. *J. Endourol.* 2013; 27: 715-21.
[29] Seitz C, Tanovic E, Kikic Z, Fajkovic H. Impact of stone size, location, composition, impaction, and hydronephrosis on the efficacy of holmium:YAG-laser ureterolithotripsy. *Eur. Urol.* 2007; 52: 1751-7.
[30] Takazawa R, Kitayama S, Tsujii T. Single-session ureteroscopy with holmium laser lithotripsy for multiple stones. *Int. J. Urol.* 2012; 19: 1118-21.
[31] Delakas D, Karyotis I, Daskalopoulos G, Lianos E, Mavromanolakis E. Independent predictors of failure of shockwave lithotripsy for ureteral stones employing a second-generation lithotripter. *J. Endourol.* 2003; 17: 201-5.
[32] Ito H, Kawahara T, Terao H, Ogawa T, Yao M, Kubota Y, et al. Predictive value of attenuation coefficients measured as Hounsfield units on noncontrast computed tomography during flexible ureteroscopy with holmium laser lithotripsy: a single-center experience. *J. Endourol.* 2012; 26: 1125-30.
[33] Pareek G, Armenakas NA, Panagopoulos G, Bruno JJ, Fracchia JA. Extracorporeal shock wave lithotripsy success based on body mass index and Hounsfield units. *Urology.* 2005; *J. Endourol. J. Endourol.* 65: 33-6.

[34] el-Assmy A, Abou-el-Ghar ME, el-Nahas AR, Refaie HF, Sheir KZ. Multidetector computed tomogr *J. E J. Endourol. ndourol.* aphy: role in determination of urinary stones composition and disintegration with extracorporeal shock wave lithotripsy--an in vitro study. *Urology.* 2011; 77: 286-90.
[35] Pareek G, Armenakas NA, Fracchia JA. Hounsfield units on computerized tomography predict stone-free rates after extracorporeal shock wave lithotripsy. *J. Urol.* 2003; 169: 1679-81.
[36] Weizer AZ, Auge BK, Silverstein AD, Delvecchio FC, Brizuela RM, Dahm P, et al. Routine postoperative imaging is important after ureteroscopic stone manipulation. *J. Urol.* 2002; 168: 46-50.
[37] Bugg CE, Jr., El-Galley R, Kenney PJ, Burns JR. Follow-up functional radiographic studies are not mandatory for all patients after ureteroscopy. *Urology.* 2002; 59: 662-7.
[38] Karadag MA, Tefekli A, Altunrende F, Tepeler A, Baykal M, Muslumanoglu AY. Is routine radiological surveillance mandatory after uncomplicated ureteroscopic stone removal? *J. Endourol.* 2008; 22: 261-6.
[39] Karod JW, Danella J, Mowad JJ. Routine radiologic surveillance for obstruction is not required in asymptomatic patients after ureteroscopy. *J. Endourol.* 1999; 13: 433-6.

Chapter 9

Complications of Ureteroscopy

Tetsuo Yoshikawa, M.D., Ph.D.*
Department of Urology, Tokyo Metropolitan Health and Medical
Treatment Corporation, Toshima Hospital, Tokyo, Japan

Abstract

Uretroscopic surgery has been established as a minimally invasive and low morbidity surgery for urinary stones and upper tract urothelial carcinoma. However, ureteroscopy is still the most common cause of ureteral injury. Most of the complications, such as mucosal abrasions and ureteral perforation after ureteroscopy, are relatively moderate and require no interventions.

The incidence of urinary tract infection after contemporary ureteroscopy has been reported to be 1.1%. Sterilizing the urine with culture-directed antibiotics prior to ureteroscopy is important, and the use of periureteroscopic antibiotics up to 24 h after the procedure is recommended.

Although the rate of complications during ureteroscopy has been decreasing as a result of improved instruments and techniques, major complications can lead to significant risk for the patients and can be challenging to manage.

---

* Corresponding author: Tetsuo Yoshikawa, M.D., Ph.D. tetsuo_yoshikawa@tokyo-hmt.jp.

Introduction

Since the first ureteroscopic study was performed by Young and Mckay in 1912, significant advances in the technology have allowed for its application in the diagnosis and treatment of urolithiasis or upper tract urothelial carcinoma. Although it can provide many therapeutic benefits, ureteroscopy may be associated with major or minor complications. Recently, complications have become less prevalent due to the miniaturization of semi-rigid and flexible ureteroscopes and the increasing experience of surgeons with ureteroscopy. However, ureteroscopy is still the most common cause of ureteral injury. Therefore, surgeons should take care to prevent potential complications and to optimize their management strategies in the event that a complication develops.

According to the EAU 2013 guidelines, complications after TUL occurred in 9-25% of the patients, most of which were not severe and required no interventions [1]. In a study of 11,885 patients by De La Rosette and associates, intraoperative complications occurred in 7.3% of the patients, including significant bleeding (1.4%), ureteral perforation or avulsion (1.1%) and failure to complete the operation (1.6%). The postoperative complication rate was low, at 3.5% of patients, and the complications included fever (1.8%) and persistent hematuria (0.4%). A blood transfusion was required in 0.2% of patients. The majority of complications were Clavien grade I or II (2.8% of patients). Five patients had a Clavien grade V event; the causes of death were sepsis, lung embolism, cardiac death, multiorgan dysfunction and sudden death from arrythmia.[2]

1. Intraoperative Complications

1.1. Mucosal Abrasion

Some degree of ureteral mucosal abrasion frequently occurs with most uretroscopic procedures. Ureteral mucosal abrasions were reported in 24% of rigid older type ureteroscopies, but only 6% of the cases using the smaller caliber newer semirigid ureteroscopes [3]. The principles for minimizing mucosal abrasion include careful technique, avoiding rough, rapid movements in the ureter and keeping the ureteral lumen in view when advancing and withdrawing the ureteroscope. The use of ureteral access sheaths when expecting multiple passes with the ureteroscope can also help minimize mucosal abrasions.

1.1. Perforation

Ureteral perforation occurs when a hole is created across all layers of the ureteral wall. The incidence of perforation has been reported to be approximately 2% or less [4]. Larger stones or impacted stones, retroperitoneal fibrosis and a prolonged operation are all associated with an increased risk of perforation.

The use of a small caliber ureteroscope and safer intraluminal lithotripters are responsible for the decreasing rate of ureteral perforation. Small ureteral perforations, such as small puncture holes induced by a guidewire or a laser fiber, are often of little consequence. Larger perforations often require further surgical repair. In all instances, ureteral stent placement and the administration of antibiotics are advised. The duration of stenting can be between one week and six weeks. Careful technique and the use of a ureteral access sheath can minimize perforation.

1.2. Avulsion

The most severe intraoperative complication of ureteroscopy is ureteral avulsion. This occurs when the ureter circumferentially tears apart, resulting in total discontinuity of the ureter. If avulsion is recognized intraoperatively, immediate surgical intervention should be performed.

Reconstruction of an avulsed ureter can be quite challenging, and may ultimately lead to a loss of affected renal function. Reconstruction can be performed by conventional open or laparoscopic surgery, and can be repaired immediately if the patient is stable. The most common cause of avulsion is attempted basket extraction of stones too large to safely pass down the ureter. The most frequent site of avulsion is the ureteropelvic junction, which can be explained by the local anatomy. Fortunately, ureteral avulsion is a rare occurrence, with a documented incidence less than 1% in most reports, and this has decreased with the increasing use of ureteroscopy [5]. The use of ureteral access sheaths has not been reported to cause ureteral avulsion.

1.3. Bleeding

Bleeding is encountered with ureteral orifice dilation or upon mucosal or calyceal injury from guidewires or ureteroscopes trauma, or during the laser destruction of renal or ureteral stones. The incidence of bleeding has been reported to be between 0.1 and 2.1%. In most of the cases, a blood transfusion was not required, and the bleeding was resolved by ureteral stent insertion [2]. In general, careful technique can help minimize potential bleeding and allow for successful ureteroscopy.

2. Early Postoperative Complications

Despite the appropriate use of preoperative antibiotics and a negative urine culture, urinary stones can harbor bacteria that may cause serious infections after lithotripsy. Pressurized irrigation can facilitate the translocation of bacteria and promote sepsis. According to the EAU 2013 guidelines, the incidence of urinary tract infection after contemporary ureteroscopy has been reported to be 1.1% [1].

Many strategies exist to reduce urinary tract infections after ureteroscopy. Sterilizing the urine with culture-directed antibiotics prior to ureteroscopy should be considered. The use of periureteroscopic antibiotics for up to 24 h is recommended by the AUA [6]. Using low pressure irrigation and only as much irrigation as necessary for adequate visualization can minimize the irrigation backflow into the renal parenchyma. Ureteral access sheaths and bladder drainage can also reduce the renal collecting system pressure and prevent subsequent microbial translocation.

3. Late Postoperative Complications

3.1. Silent Hydronephrosis

The incidence of asymptomatic or silent hydronephrosis after ureteroscopy has been reported to be 4.8% [7]. These patients have ongoing silent obstruction that may eventually lead to the loss of renal function of the affected kidney. Routine imaging after uncomplicated ureteroscopy may not be necessary in asymptomatic patients. However, after complicated ureteroscopy, such as in cases with impacted stones, postoperative pain, intraoperative ureteral injury or after ureteral balloon dilation, routine imaging after the operation should be mandatory. If a hydronephrosis is detected by ultrasound or non-contrast computed tomography, further functional imaging and diagnostic studies can be considered.

3.2. Ureteral Stricture

The incidence of ureteral stricture after routine ureteroscopy is between 0 and 4% [8]. The exact etiology of stricture formation is unclear, but may be a combination of direct instrument trauma, thermal injury and possibly relative ischemia from larger diameter instruments. In addition, an impacted ureteral stone which is embedded within the ureteral wall may predispose to granuloma formation and subsequent ureteral stricture. Patients with upper tract urothelial carcinoma managed primary by ureteroscopy appear to be at higher risk than those undergoing ureteroscopy for urinary stones. The reasons include the use of repeated screening, direct laser ablation of ureteral tissue and upper tract BCG exposure. Recurrent strictures, long strictures and segments with multiple strictures are usually repaired by conventional open or laparoscopic surgery.

Conclusion

Ureteroscopic surgery has made it possible to perform minimally invasive surgery for urinary stones and upper tract urothelial carcinoma with low morbidity. To achieve safe and successful operations, surgeons should understand the possible complications, and develop strategies to manage the complications if they arise.

References

[1] European Association of Urology (EAU) Guidelines. Guidelines on urolithiasis. EAU 2013.

[2] De La Rosette J, Denstedt J, Geavlete P, et al. The clinical research office of the endourological society ureteroxcopy global study:

indications, complications, and outcomes in 11,885 patients. *J. Endourol.* 2014; 28: 131-9.

[3] Francesca F, Scattoni V, Nava L, et al. Failures and complications of transurethral ureteroscopy in 297 cases: conventional rigid instruments vs small caliber semirigid ureteroscopes. *Eur. Urol.* 1995; 28: 112-5.

[4] Geavlete P, Georgescu D, Nita G, et al. Complications of 2735 retrograde semirigid uretroscopy procedures: a single-center experience. *J. Endourol.* 2006; 20: 179-85.

[5] Stoller ML, Wolf JS. Endoscopic ureteral injuries. In: McAninch JW, editor. Traumatic and reconstructive urology. 1996; Philadelphia: WB Saunders; P. 199-211.

[6] Wolf Jr JS, Bennett CJ, Dmochowski RR, et al. Urologic surgery antimicrobial prophylaxis best practice policy panel. Best practice policy statement on urologic surgery antimicrobial prophylaxis. *J. Urol.* 2008; 179: 1379-90.

[7] Manger JP, Mendoza PJ, Babayan RK, et al. Use of renal ultrasound to detect hydronephrosis after ureteroscopy. *J. Endourol.* 2009; 23: 1399-402.

[8] Johnson DB, Pearle MS. Complications of ureteroscopy. *Urol. Clin. North Am.* 2004; 31: 157-71.

Chapter 10

Evidence for Staged Operations

Ryoji Takazawa[*], *M.D., Ph.D., Sachi Kitayama, M.D.
and Toshihiko Tsujii, M.D., Ph.D.*
Department of Urology, Tokyo Metropolitan Ohtsuka Hospital,
Tokyo, Japan

Abstract

Thanks to the recent advances in endoscopic technology, ureteroscopy (URS) has become a more efficient and safer treatment option for stones throughout the entire urinary collecting system. Percutaneous nephrolithotomy (PNL) is currently the first-line recommended treatment for patients with renal stones larger than 2 cm. PNL has an excellent success rate in clearing large renal stones. However, its invasiveness cannot be overlooked considering the relatively low, but not negligible, major complication rates. Staged URS is a practical option for the treatment of large renal stones. Staged URS is associated with a minimal blood transfusion risk, short hospitalization and few restrictions on daily routines, which allows patients to work between procedures. However, as the treated stone grows larger in size, the success rate of URS monotherapy decreases, and the number of procedures required increases. Therefore, in our opinion, PNL should be considered preferentially for stones larger than 4 cm. However, URS is an

---

[*] Corresponding author: Ryoji Takazawa, M.D., Ph.D. ryoji_takazawa@tmhp.jp.

efficient treatment for multiple upper urinary tract stones. For patients with a stone burden < 20 mm, either unilaterally or bilaterally, URS is a favorable option that promises a high stone-free rate after a single session. However, for patients with a stone burden ≥ 20 mm, a staged operation should be considered to achieve stone-free status.

Introduction

Thanks to the recent advances in endoscopic technology, ureteroscopy (URS) has become a more efficient and safer treatment for stones throughout the entire urinary collecting system. In this chapter, we discuss the possibilities and limitations of ureteroscopic lithotripsy in terms of the stone size and stone number.

1. Large Renal Stones

Percutaneous nephrolithotomy (PNL) is currently the recommended first-line treatment for patients with renal stones larger than 2 cm [1, 2]. PNL has an excellent success rate in clearing large renal stones. However, its invasiveness cannot be overlooked considering the relatively low, but not negligible, major complication rates. Renal parenchymal damage is inevitable in PNL, and its major complications are usually related to the puncture or dilation of a nephrostomy tract. A recent global study of PNL reported the major complication rates, including 7.8% of cases experiencing significant bleeding, 3.4% experiencing renal pelvis perforation and 1.8% developing hydrothorax [3]. Blood transfusions were necessary in 5.7% of cases, and a high-grade fever occurred in 10.5% of the patients. The use of the prone position during the procedure also increases the anesthetic risks.

Recently, flexible URS has become a more efficient and safer treatment for stones throughout all renal calyces. URS is an endoscopic surgery performed through the natural orifice, thus, renal parenchymal damage can be avoided. The ureteroscopes and their working devices have rapidly improved over the past few years. Retrograde URS with holmium laser lithotripsy results in an equivalent or superior result to shock wave lithotripsy (SWL) for ureteral stones, as well as small renal stones [1, 2]. Several single institution case series of URS for large renal stones have been reported. In 1998, Grasso et al. reported that 45 patients with renal stones larger than 2 cm underwent URS, with a 76% stone-free rate after a single procedure. Second stage procedures were carried out in 15 patients, and the success rate increased to 91% without intraoperative complications [4]. This remarkable result was followed by additional reports [5-8] with similar findings.

We previously reported an overall 90% stone-free rate for an average stone size of 3.1 cm with an average 1.4 procedures [9]. In particular, in a subset of 14 patients with stones 2 to 4 cm, we satisfactorily achieved a 100% stone-free rate that included 64% (9/14) of cases with no residual fragments. Our stone-free rate after a second URS is promising and equivalent to that of PNL. In our study, three patients (15%) developed a postoperative high-grade fever despite the administration of antibiotics that were specific for the detected bacteria. One patient, who had no comorbidities, developed sepsis after the first procedure. She had a struvite stone and the intraoperative visualization was poor as a result of the snow storm caused by fragmentation. It is impossible to completely avoid postoperative infections because of the spread of bacteria from infectious stones into the irrigation fluid during fragmentation. Thus, a good irrigation system is important to keep the proper drainage flow and low intrarenal pressure, as well as the administration of antibiotics. A long operation also apparently increases complication rates. If we cannot finish within 120 mines, we usually consider performing a staged operation.

Consequently, staged URS is a practical option for the treatment of large renal stones. Staged URS has little blood transfusion risk, is associated with a short hospitalization and few restrictions on daily routines, which allows patients to work between procedures. Furthermore, the latest digital ureteroscopes have excellent image quality and easy handling, promising better outcomes in the near future [10]. However, as the treated stone grows larger in size, the success rate of URS monotherapy decreases, and the number of procedures increases. In our study, the stone free rate for stones > 4 cm decreased to 67% after an average of 1.8 procedures, compared with a 100% stone-free rate for stones 2 to 4 cm by an average of 1.3 procedures [9]. Therefore, in our opinion, PNL should be considered preferentially for stones larger than 4 cm.

Recently, the new technique of "miniperc" or "tubeless PNL," which utilizes a smaller caliber nephrostomy tract, was developed, and is expected to decrease the risk of perioperative complications [11]. This new less-invasive PNL has the possibility of replacing conventional PNL for the treatment of very large stone burdens, including complete staghorn calculi. Furthermore, a synchronous approach with URS and PNL in the Galdakao-modified supine

Valdivia position has been reported, and is expected to be superior to PNL monotherapy [12].

2. Multiple Stones

Multiple stones are found in 20–25% of patients with urolithiasis [13–15]. The stone-free rates for patients with multiple stones after SWL are reported to be 40–50%, which is significantly lower than that for patients with a single stone [13, 16]. The stone number (single *vs* multiple) was a powerful predictor influencing the treatment outcome after SWL in the multivariate analyses [2, 13–15, 17]. Recently, retrograde URS has become an effective and safe treatment for either renal or ureteral stones, and its indications have been expanding [18–20]. The advantages of URS over SWL are its ability to directly access stones throughout the entire urinary collecting system either unilaterally or bilaterally, and to actively remove stone fragments. Thus, for multiple stones, URS is likely an ideal treatment that promises a high stone-free rate after a single session.

SWL has been accepted as the first-line treatment for small (< 10 mm) to moderate sized (<20 mm) upper urinary tract stones [2]. The advantages of SWL are patient acceptance, short convalescence and the lack of a requirement for anesthesia during the procedure. However, many factors (the stone location, size, number, composition and the patient's body mass index) influence the outcome [13–17]. In particular, the stone multiplicity is one of the adverse factors associated with the stone-free rates and/or recurrence-free rates after SWL. In 2005, Abe et al. reported that the stone-free rate for multiple stones was just 41% (231/569 patients) compared with 71% (1763/2492 patients) for single stones [13]. The stone number (single *vs* multiple) was the most significant predictor for recurrence in the multivariate analyses.

PNL is another option for the treatment of multiple renal stones. Multiple stones sometimes necessitate multiple access tracts, which increase the risk of complications and the patient's discomfort.

Flexible ureteroscopes and their working devices have rapidly improved over the past few years. URS now leads to an equivalent or superior result to SWL for renal stones, as well as ureteral stones [2, 18]. URS has some advantages for the treatment of multiple stones compared with SWL and PNL. First, URS can actively remove the stone fragments by using a nitinol basket, and can continue the fragmentation of the other stones in a single session. Second, the latest flexible ureteroscopes can approach all calyces, including the lower calyx, where residual fragments after SWL are difficult to pass spontaneously and often lead to recurrent stone formation. Third, URS can easily access bilateral stones in a single session.

There have been some reports on the ureteroscopic management of multiple stones [21, 22]. For example, Breda et al. reported their experiences with 51 patients who had multiple unilateral renal stones [21]. For 24 patients with a renal stone burden ≤ 20 mm, the stone-free rate after one and two procedures was 79% and 100%, respectively, compared with 52% and 85% for 27 patients with a renal stone burden > 20 mm. We previously reported a study where, although both renal and ureteral stones (unilateral or bilateral) were included in the study cohort, the treatment results were comparable with those in Breda's reports [23]. Furthermore, we showed that the "stone burden" and the presence of "impacted stones" were significant predictors of the stone-free rate after a single session URS, whereas the stone locations did not strongly influence the treatment outcome. For "impacted stones", when the ureteral mucosa was widely damaged during lithotripsy, we interrupted the procedure to avoid a risk of ureteral stricture and left a ureteral stent to prepare for a second session for residual stones. In our study, we carried out 14 simultaneous bilateral URS procedures with no complications, and achieved stone-free status after a single session in 12 patients. The safety and efficacy of a simultaneous bilateral URS has been reported by some experts [24, 25]. Our results further reinforce that a simultaneous bilateral URS is a favorable option for bilateral stones in experienced institutions.

We also reported our surgical outcome data, both overall and comparing patients with a stone burden < 20 mm and ≥ 20 mm [23]. Overall, the mean number of procedures per patient was 1.3 ± 0.6. The mean total length of the operation per patient was 112 ± 70 min (median 88, range 27–375). Overall, the stone-free rate after one and two procedures was 80.4% (41/51) and 92.2% (47/51), respectively. The 25 patients with a stone burden < 20 mm underwent a significantly smaller number of procedures, had a shorter total length of the operation(s) and had a higher stone-free rate after the first procedure than the 26 patients with a stone burden ≥ 20 mm, although the stone-free rates after the second procedure were not significantly different. No major intraoperative complications, including ureteral perforation, were identified. A postoperative high-grade fever >38.5°C was observed after three procedures in three patients, who were all conservatively cured by the administration of antibiotics.

Consequently, URS is an efficient treatment for multiple upper urinary tract stones. For patients with a stone burden < 20 mm, either unilaterally or bilaterally, URS is a favorable option that promises a high stone-free rate after a single session. However, for patients with a stone burden ≥ 20 mm, a staged operation should be considered to achieve a stone-free status.

Conclusion

For large renal stones, staged URS is a practical option for treatment. Staged URS is associated with a minimal risk of needing a blood transfusion, short hospitalization and few restrictions on daily routines, which allows patients to work between procedures. However, as the treated stone grows larger in size, the success rate of URS monotherapy decreases, and the number of procedures increases. Therefore, in our opinion, PNL should be considered preferentially for stones larger than 4 cm.

In addition, URS is an efficient treatment for multiple upper urinary tract stones. For patients with a stone burden < 20 mm, either unilaterally or bilaterally, URS is a favorable option that promises a high stone-free rate after a single session.

References

[1] Lingeman J, Matlaga B, Evan A. Surgical management of upper urinary tract calculi. In: Wein AJ, Kavoussi LR, Novick AC, Partin AW, Peters CA (eds). *Cambell-Walsh Urology*, 9th edn. Saunders Elsevier, Philadelphia, PA; 1437–1438, 2007.

[2] European Association of Urology (EAU) Guidelines. Guidelines on urolithiasis. EAU, Arnhem, 2011.

[3] de la Rosette J, Assimos D, Desai M et al. The clinical research office of the endourological society percutaneous nephrolithotomy global study: indications, complications, and outcomes in 5803 patients. *J. Endourol.* 2011;25: 11–17.

[4] Grasso M, Conlin M, Bagley D. Retrograde ureteropyeloscopic treatment of 2 cm or greater upper urinary tract and minor staghorn calculi. *J. Urol.* 1998; 160: 346–51.

[5] Breda A, Ogunyemi O, Leppert JT, Lam JS, Schulam PG. Flexible ureteroscopy and laser lithotripsy for intrarenal stones 2 cm or greater – Is this the new frontier? *J. Urol.* 2008; 179: 981–84.

[6] Riley JM, Stearman L, Troxel S. Retrograde ureteroscopy for renal stones larger than 2.5 cm. *J. Endourol.* 2009; 23: 1395–1398.

[7] Ricchiuti DJ, Smaldone MC, Jacobs BL, Smaldone AM, Jackman SV, Averch TD. Staged retrograde endoscopic lithotripsy as alternative to PCNL in select patients with large renal calculi. *J. Endourol.* 2007; 21: 1421–24.

[8] Hyams ES, Munver R, Bird VG, Uberoi J, Shah O. Flexible ureteroscopy and holmium laser lithotripsy for the management of renal stone burdens that measure 2 to 3 cm: a multi – institutional experience. *J. Endourol.* 2010; 24: 1583–88.

[9] Takazawa R, Kitayama S, Tsujii T. Successful outcome of flexible ureteroscopy with holmium laser lithotripsy for renal stones 2 cm or greater. *Int. J. Urol.* 2012; 19: 264–67.

[10] Humphreys MR, Miller NL, Williams JC, Evan AP, Munch LC, Lingeman JE. A new world revealed: early experience with digital ureteroscopy. *J. Urol.* 2008; 179: 970–75.

[11] Jackmann SV, Docimo SG, Cadeddu JA et al. The "miniperc" technique: a less invasive alternative to percutaneous nephrolithotomy. *World J. Urol.* 1998; 16: 371–74.

[12] Scoffone CM, Cracco CM, Cossu M, Grande S, Paggio M, Scarpa RM. Endoscopic combined intrarenal surgery in Galdakao-modified supine Valdivia position: a new standard for percutaneous nephrolithotomy? *Eur. Urol.* 2008; 54: 1393–403.

[13] Abe T, Akakura K, Kawaguchi M et al. Outcomes of shockwave lithotripsy for upper urinary tract stones: a large-scale study at a single institution. *J. Endourol.* 2005; 19: 768 73.

[14] Kanao K, Nakashima J, Nakagawa K et al. Preoperative nomograms for predicting stone-free rate after extracorporeal shock wave lithotripsy. *J. Urol.* 2006; 176: 1453–57.

[15] Abdel-Khalek M, Sheir KZ, Mokhtar AA, Eraky I, Kenawy M, Bazeed M. Prediction of success rate after extracorporeal shock-wave lithotripsy of renal stones- a multivariate analysis model. *Scand. J. Urol. Nephrol.* 2004; 38: 161–67.

[16] Cass AS. Comparison of first generation (Dornier HM3) and second generation (Medstone STS) lithotripters: treatment results with 13,864 renal and ureteral calculi. *J. Urol.* 1995; 153: 588–92.

[17] El-Assmy A, El-Nahas AR, Abo-Elghar ME, Eraky I, El-Kenawy MR, Sheir KZ. Predictors of success after extracorporeal shock wave lithotripsy (ESWL) for renal calculi between 20–30 mm: a multivariate analysis model. *Scientific World Journal* 2006; 6: 2388–90.
[18] Galvin DJ, Pearle MS. The contemporary management of renal and ureteric calculi. *BJU Int.* 2006; 98: 1283–88.
[19] Anagnostou T, Tolley D. Management of ureteric stones. *Eur. Urol.* 2004; 45: 714–21.
[20] Takazawa R, Kitayama S, Kobayashi S et al. Transurethral lithotripsy with rigid and flexible ureteroscopy for renal and ureteral stones: results of the first 100 procedures. *Hinyokika Kiyo* 2011; 57: 411–16.
[21] Breda A, Ogunyemi O, Leppert JT, Schulam PG. Flexible ureteroscopy and laser lithotripsy for multiple unilateral intrarenal stones. *Eur. Urol.* 2009; 55: 1190–97.
[22] Herrera-Gonzalez G, Netsch C, Oberhagemann K, Bach T, Gross AJ. Effectiveness of single flexible ureteroscopy for multiple renal calculi. *J. Endourol.* 2011; 25: 431–35.
[23] Takazawa R, Kitayama S, Tsujii T. Single-session ureteroscopy with holmium laser lithotripsy for multiple stones. *Int. J. Urol.* 2012; 19: 1118–21.
[24] Hollenbeck BK, Schuster TG, Faeber GJ, Wolf S. Safety and efficacy of same-session bilateral ureteroscopy. *J. Endourol.* 2004; 17: 881–85.
[25] Watson JM, Chang C, Pattaras JG, Ogan K. Same session bilateral ureteroscopy is safe and efficacious. *J. Urol.* 2011; 185: 170–74.

POSTFACE: FUTURE VISION

Over the past two decades, ureteroscopy has undergone a remarkable evolution. In particular, the recent developments of smaller, more flexible ureteroscopes, higher-resolution cameras and a wide variety of novel instruments have changed the treatment options for urolithiasis. The treatment choice has shifted from shock-wave lithotripsy to ureteroscopic lithotripsy. Ureteroscopy has also improved the outcome of percutaneous nephrolithotomy when it is used in a combination procedure. However, there are still some issues that need to be resolved.

Several digital ureteroscopes have been introduced over the past few years. The biggest benefit of a digital ureteroscope is its excellent imaging capabilities. The image is much larger and clearer than that provided by a fiberoptic ureteroscope. In contrast, one of the disadvantages of the digital ureteroscopes available today are their larger tip size and higher cost than fiberoptic ureteroscopes. The tip size has been evolving to be smaller while maintaining its high-resolution image. We expect it to become as small as 7 or 8 Fr, which is the same as fiberoptic ureteroscopes.

Fiberoptic ureteroscopes have also advanced in terms of their size, performance and durability. The current smallest tip is 5.3 Fr. The smaller tip design makes it easier to insert into the narrow ureter. The size of the ureteral access sheath can also be decreased. Future studies should investigate the appropriate combination of a ureteroscope and ureteral access sheath that can optimize the visualization, irrigation flow and easy retrieval of stone fragments. Most of the fiberoptic ureteroscopes available today have only one channel. Two-channel ureteroscopes would enable more sophisticated intrarenal surgery in the future.

The application of a holmium:YAG laser remains the most common mode of fragmentation during ureteroscopy. Although the holmium:YAG laser has ideal properties for ureteroscopic treatment, the fragments are sometimes too small to extract. Currently, we repeat the retrieval of stone fragments using a basket catheter many times. Otherwise, the stones can be broken up by the "dust technique" with low energy (0.2-0.5 J) and high frequency (20-50 Hz), which makes the stone fragments very small, so that it is unnecessary to extract them. We expect a more effective method to be developed. One of the ideas is the magnetic extraction of stone fragments [1-3]. The new technology is now in the proof-of-concept stage, with further work needed to improve its reliability and ensure its safety in humans.

A robotic system for flexible ureteroscopic surgery has been developed. The Sensei® robotic catheter system has been applied to ureteroscopic surgery. The system was initially developed for cardiovascular applications, such as endocardial ablation for arrhythmia. The system's hardware and software have been adapted and modified for ureteroscopy [4, 5]. The new technology has the potential to provide improved precision, better ergonomics and reduced occupational radiation exposure. Further studies are necessary to determine if there is a clinical advantage, and if the benefits outweigh the potentially increased cost of the system.

The ureteroscopic training for young urologists should be better organized. Some critical complications, including ureteral avulsion and postoperative ureteral stricture, must be avoided. There are some high-fidelity simulators for ureteroscopic surgery. These are constructed using materials such as latex and silicone to replicate human tissues, and often employ the use of standard endoscopic equipment [6, 7]. Significant advances in available materials have allowed more accurate representations, allowing for a more realistic simulation experience. Trainees should learn the basic manipulation of ureteroscopes by using simulators.

In conclusion, we expect that future technical advancements will be able to resolve the above-mentioned issues, and believe that ureteroscopic surgery will become more sophisticated in the near future.

Ryoji Takazawa, M.D., Ph.D.

References

[1] Tracy CR, Mcleroy SL, Best SL, Gnade BE, Pearle MS, Cadeddu JA. Rendering stone fragments paramagnetic with iron-oxide microparticles improves the efficiency and effectiveness of endoscopic stone fragment retrieval. *Urology.* 76: 2010; 5: 1266e10-4.

[2] Mir SA, Best SL, Mcleroy SL, et al. Novel stone-magnetizing microparticles: in vitro toxicity and biologic functionality analysis. *J. Endourol.* 2011; 25: 1203-7.

[3] Tan YK, McLeroy SL, Faddegon S, et al. In vitro comparison of prototype magnetic tool with conventional nitinol basket for ureteroscopic retrieval of stone fragments rendered paramagnetic with iron oxide microparticles. *J. Urol.* 2012; 188: 648-52.

[4] Desai MM, Aron M, Gill IS, et al. Flexible robotic retrograde renoscopy: description of novel robotic device and preliminary laboratory experience. *Urology.* 2008; 71: 42-6.

[5] Desai MM, Grover R, Aron M, et al. Robotic flexible ureteroscopy for renal calculi: initial clinical experience. *J. Urol.* 2011; 186: 563-8.

[6] White MA, Dehaan AP, Stephens DD, et al. Validation of a high fidelity adult ureteroscopy and renoscopy simulator. *J. Urol.* 2010; 183: 673-7.

[7] Watterson JD, Denstedt JD. Ureteroscopy and cystoscopy simulation in urology. *J. Endourol.* 2007; 21: 263-9.

Authors' Contact Information

Dr. Ryoji Takazawa
Department of Urology
Tokyo Metropolitan Ohtsuka Hospital
2-8-1 Toshima-ku, Minami-Ohtsuka
170-8476 Tokyo, Japan
Tel: +81-3-3941-3211
E-mail: ryoji_takazawa@tmhp.jp

Dr. Sachi Kitayama
Department of Urology
Tokyo Metropolitan Ohtsuka Hospital
2-8-1 Toshima-ku, Minami-Ohtsuka
170-8476 Tokyo, Japan

Dr. Toshihiko Tsujii
Department of Urology
Tokyo Metropolitan Ohtsuka Hospital
2-8-1 Toshima-ku, Minami-Ohtsuka
170-8476 Tokyo, Japan

Dr. Junichi Matsuzaki
Department of Urology
Ohguchi Higashi Genaral Hospital
Yokohama, Japan

Dr. Takashi Kawahara
Department of Urology
Ohguchi Higashi Genaral Hospital
Yokohama, Japan

Dr. Hiroki Ito
Department of Urology
Ohguchi Higashi Genaral Hospital
Yokohama, Japan

Dr. Tetsuo Yoshikawa
Department of Urology
Tokyo Metropolitan Health and Medical Treatment Corporation
Toshima Hospital,
Tokyo, Japan

Index

A

acute renal failure, 59
AD, 95, 125
adhesion, 104
adsorption, 97
adults, 46, 109
advancement(s), 32, 142
adverse effects, 34
adverse event, 37, 38
aetiology, 16
age, 56, 88
algorithm, 8, 9, 10, 12
amplitude, 48
anastomosis, 43
anatomy, 15, 49, 79, 81, 106, 129
anesthesiologist, 73, 75
antibiotic, 54, 55, 59, 60, 97
anticoagulation, 12
arrhythmia, 142
arteriography, 46
assessment, 60, 113, 116, 122, 123
asymptomatic, 4, 5, 13, 14, 46, 120, 125, 130
avulsion, 32, 72, 128, 129, 142

B

bacteria, 90, 130, 135
bending, 82
benefits, 36, 142
benign, 91
biliary tract, 46
biocompatible materials, 44
biomaterials, 44
bleeding, 12, 41, 80, 128, 130, 134
blends, 44
blood, 35, 37, 47, 128, 130, 133, 135, 138
blood flow, 35, 47
blood transfusion, 128, 130, 133, 135, 138
BMI, 115
body mass index, 12, 107, 124, 136
brittleness, 44
burn, 24

C

calcium, 12, 38, 39, 91
calcium channel blocker, 38
calculus, 15, 21, 32, 105, 106, 108, 116
caliber, 23, 29, 32, 46, 91, 128, 129, 132, 135
calyx, 3, 7, 8, 15, 30, 40, 41, 72, 74, 79, 82, 83, 101, 104, 106, 109, 137
cancer, 68
candidates, 55, 106, 115
carcinoma, 21, 127, 128, 131
catastrophic failure, 25

catecholamines, 37
catheter, 21, 29, 34, 46, 47, 56, 57, 65, 66, 80, 83, 84, 85, 86, 90, 93, 94, 101, 103, 106, 142
cefazolin, 54, 60
children, 58, 60, 115
City, 53, 77, 87, 99, 113
cladding, 21
classification, 86
clinical trials, 43
coatings, 45, 55, 88
colic, 5, 88, 115, 116, 123
collagen, 36
combination therapy, 114
complications, 8, 31, 44, 47, 49, 53, 54, 56, 59, 62, 64, 67, 75, 84, 85, 89, 90, 92, 94, 100, 102, 103, 105, 106, 107, 114, 121, 127, 128, 131, 132, 134, 135, 136, 137, 138, 142
composition, 7, 12, 37, 86, 124, 125, 136
computed tomography, 57, 90, 113, 114, 123, 124, 131
configuration, 23, 25
congestive heart failure, 37
consensus, 4
construction, 20
controlled trials, 44, 54
controversial, 44
correlation(s), 56, 57, 89, 90, 91, 93
correlation coefficient, 57, 90
cost, 35, 92, 141, 142
crochet hook, 92, 97
CSD, 118
CT, 12, 57, 68, 90, 93, 101, 114, 115, 116, 122, 123
CT scan, 12, 68, 101, 115, 122
culture, 12, 127, 130
cysteine, 12, 39
cystine, 80
cystoscopy, 63, 64, 65, 78, 85, 92, 93, 97, 106, 143

D

danger, 104

database, 34
degradation, 21, 40, 68
demographic data, 34
deposition, 36
depth, 73
destruction, 130
detectable, 121
detection, 25, 68, 114
detection system, 25
digital ureteroscope, 25, 29, 135, 141
dilation, 22, 32, 43, 44, 47, 60, 72, 100, 102, 103, 105, 130, 131, 134
direct measure, 57, 89, 90
discomfort, 45, 55, 88, 136
discontinuity, 129
disease progression, 5
displacement, 43, 47, 83
distribution, 11
donors, 34
double ureter, 109
drainage, 12, 34, 43, 44, 45, 59, 78, 100, 102, 130, 135
durability, 25, 40, 68, 81, 141
dysuria, 45

E

edema, 34, 88
education, 13
electrolyte, 37
electrolyte imbalance, 37
embolism, 128
emergency, 43, 44, 93, 122
EMS, 101
endoscope, 25, 34, 36, 39, 68, 78, 80
endoscopy, 20, 35, 36, 37, 38
energy, 36, 38, 39, 40, 68, 80, 84, 142
engineering, 61, 95
environment, 38, 44
epinephrine, 38
equipment, 20, 65, 78, 84, 142
ergonomics, 142
etiology, 121, 131
evidence, 36, 43, 83
evolution, 4, 20, 141

exclusion, 102
excretion, 80, 83
exercise, 64
experimental condition, 35
exposure, 100, 131, 142
expulsion, 13, 71
extraction, 31, 40, 41, 60, 75, 80, 83, 85, 95, 102, 129, 142
extravasation, 37, 44

F

fat, 101
fetus, 116
fever, 44, 54, 103, 128, 134, 135, 137
fiber(s), 21, 22, 23, 24, 25, 38, 39, 46, 66, 67, 68, 73, 78, 80, 83, 84, 129
fiberoptic, 19, 21, 22, 23, 24, 25, 27, 29, 67, 86, 141
fidelity, 142, 143
filiform, 40
films, 115
fires, 25
first generation, 139
flank, 43, 58, 59, 114, 122, 123
flexibility, 19, 21, 23, 24, 29, 31, 39, 41, 44, 78, 83
flexible ureteroscope, 21, 22, 23, 24, 25, 27, 28, 30, 32, 34, 37, 40, 41, 43, 67, 68, 70, 72, 77, 79, 80, 81, 83, 128, 137, 141
fluid, 34, 36, 37, 38, 82, 84, 135
force, 32, 72, 81
formation, 3, 7, 8, 12, 15, 46, 90, 92, 96, 97, 105, 131, 137
formula, 61, 96
fragility, 117
fragments, vii, 3, 7, 8, 12, 31, 32, 39, 40, 41, 44, 63, 64, 68, 74, 75, 80, 82, 83, 84, 87, 88, 117, 120, 121, 135, 136, 141, 142, 143
friction, 32
functional imaging, 121, 131
fusion, 104

G

Galdakao-modified supine Valdivia position, 14, 65, 75, 107, 136, 139
gel, 92
general anesthesia, 12, 64, 73, 78
Germany, 79, 101
gravity, 36
growth, 4
guidance, 32, 40, 67, 80, 84, 92, 97, 100, 101, 102, 104
guidelines, 7, 8, 12, 13, 59, 90, 117, 128, 130
guidewire, 29, 30, 31, 32, 57, 63, 64, 65, 66, 67, 69, 70, 71, 72, 75, 86, 90, 93, 101, 105, 129

H

hazards, 38
height, 57, 61, 89, 96
hematuria, 58, 128
history, 4, 5, 13, 19, 40, 46, 102, 104, 106
HIV, 114
holmium, 14, 19, 20, 38, 41, 48, 60, 63, 64, 67, 75, 78, 85, 86, 117, 122, 124, 134, 139, 140, 142
hospitalization, 133, 135, 138
human, 37, 142
Hunter, 100, 102, 106, 107
hybrid, 23
hydronephrosis, 43, 55, 62, 72, 82, 86, 88, 93, 105, 106, 107, 116, 117, 120, 121, 123, 124, 130, 132
hydrophilic materials, 31
hyponatremia, 37
hypothermia, 37

I

iatrogenic, 30, 67
ideal, vii, 29, 38, 57, 61, 80, 89, 96, 104, 105, 106, 136, 142
identification, 70, 114

ileal conduit, 106, 109
iliac crest, 80
illumination, 20
image(s), 21, 22, 23, 24, 25, 79, 81, 115, 135, 141
imaging modalities, 114, 115, 123
improvements, vii, 40, 78, 81
in vitro, 125, 143
in vivo, 37, 38, 97
incidence, 53, 54, 55, 56, 59, 88, 89, 91, 92, 93, 100, 103, 105, 120, 121, 127, 129, 130, 131
infection, 4, 5, 12, 44, 54, 59, 82
inflammation, 36
informed consent, 102
infundibulum, 7, 30, 72
injury(ies), 22, 32, 65, 67, 68, 72, 79, 86, 94, 101, 104, 116, 127, 128, 130, 131, 132
insertion, 21, 32, 35, 43, 44, 54, 57, 64, 65, 66, 67, 72, 79, 82, 85, 86, 91, 101, 103, 106, 130
institutions, 137
internalization, 25
intervention, 4, 5, 6, 12, 13, 114, 120, 121
iodinated contrast, 114
ionizing radiation, 115
ions, 91
ipsilateral, 46, 65
iron, 143
irrigation, 19, 21, 22, 23, 24, 31, 32, 34, 35, 36, 37, 38, 40, 41, 43, 47, 58, 66, 68, 80, 82, 84, 130, 135, 141
irrigation system, 19, 36, 37, 135
ischemia, 35, 81, 88, 131
issues, 35, 141, 142

J

Japan, 3, 19, 63, 79, 127, 133
Japanese women, 79

K

kidney(s), 3, 4, 5, 6, 8, 9, 14, 15, 29, 32, 34, 40, 43, 45, 57, 70, 73, 75, 80, 81, 82, 90, 104, 105, 107, 108, 109, 130
kidney stone(s), 3, 4, 5, 8, 9, 14, 15, 43, 81

L

laparoscopic surgery, 129, 131
laser ablation, 131
laser fiber, 23, 24, 25, 39, 40, 66, 67, 68, 73, 129
lasers, 39, 83, 87
lead, vii, 3, 7, 8, 24, 30, 32, 36, 40, 68, 72, 81, 127, 129, 130, 137
LED, 25, 29
legs, 64
lens, 19, 21, 22, 23, 24
light, 20, 21, 23, 25, 29, 64, 68
light transmission, 21
lithotripsy, vii, 3, 4, 12, 13, 14, 15, 16, 19, 38, 39, 47, 48, 54, 55, 58, 60, 63, 64, 67, 73, 75, 78, 80, 82, 83, 85, 86, 88, 93, 94, 107, 108, 117, 120, 122, 124, 125, 130, 134, 137, 139, 140, 141
liver, 101
low-dose NCCT, 121
lumen, 29, 128

M

magnesium, 91
magnetic resonance, 116
magnetic resonance imaging, 116
majority, 32, 41, 68, 117, 128
management, vii, 3, 4, 13, 14, 16, 24, 47, 59, 62, 78, 85, 86, 87, 88, 90, 96, 106, 108, 113, 115, 116, 121, 122, 124, 128, 137, 138, 139, 140
manipulation, 48, 60, 65, 78, 100, 125, 142
materials, 20, 45, 55, 88, 142
materials science, 20
matrix, 21, 91

matter, 47
measurement(s), 12, 56, 57, 61, 89, 96, 120, 122, 124
median, 56, 70, 88, 91, 93, 102, 120, 137
medical, 5, 43
medication, 12
memory, 30
meta-analysis, 8, 11, 44, 49
microparticles, 143
migration, 39, 45, 56, 61, 80, 85, 89, 90, 92, 95
miniaturization, 77, 78, 128
morbidity, 4, 12, 62, 81, 97, 103, 127, 131
morphology, 29
mortality, 103
MR, 47, 86, 107, 123, 139, 140
mucosa, 71, 79, 80, 92, 137
mucosal abrasion, 127, 128
multivariate analysis, 139, 140
muscarinic receptor, 37
muscle relaxation, 64

N

necrosis, 36
negative effects, 4
negotiating, 44
nephrolithiasis, 13, 123, 124
nephron, 103, 105, 106
next generation, 41
nickel, 30, 41, 83
nocturia, 56, 88
norepinephrine, 37, 47

O

obesity, 103
obstruction, 4, 6, 12, 29, 30, 43, 46, 54, 59, 66, 71, 106, 116, 117, 120, 121, 123, 125, 130
obstructive uropathy, 123
occlusion, 34, 47, 85, 106
OH, 38
operations, 19, 37, 131

optical fiber, 24
optical systems, 19
organs, 20, 104
outpatient, 60, 92
oxalate, 12, 39, 80

P

pain, 4, 6, 43, 45, 49, 55, 58, 59, 92, 93, 94, 114, 115, 121, 122, 123, 131
parenchyma, 101, 116, 130
participants, 102
pathology, 67, 68
pelvis, 21, 22, 34, 37, 41, 56, 79, 80, 82, 83, 89, 100, 105, 109, 134
perforation, 38, 43, 64, 67, 84, 127, 128, 129, 134, 137
perfusion, 35, 38, 47, 48
peristalsis, 38
permit, 29, 38
pH, 91
Philadelphia, 132, 138
phosphate, 39
Physiological, 37
pigs, 48
pleural cavity, 101
pneumothorax, 105
policy, 132
polymer(s), 31, 44, 60, 95
polyurethane, 44, 96
population, 61, 96, 104, 123
pregnancy, 123, 124
preparation, 54, 100, 102, 103
prestenting, 53, 55, 58, 60
prevention, 16, 59
principles, 128
prophylactic, 5, 14, 54
prophylaxis, 59, 60, 132
protection, 25
prototype, 143
PTFE, 31, 65, 70
PTFE-coated stiff guidewire, 70
pyelonephritis, 43
pyuria, 55

Q

quality of life, 5, 49, 58
questionnaire, 56, 88

R

radiation, 57, 84, 89, 100, 115, 123, 142
radical cystectomy, 106
radiography, 122
radiopaque, 115, 121
receptors, 37
recurrence, 83, 114, 136
reintroduction, 67
reliability, 57, 89, 117, 142
renal calculi, 6, 15, 34, 47, 86, 104, 139, 140, 143
renal dysfunction, 4
renal failure, 121
repair, 81, 129
requirements, 43
resistance, 41, 67, 68, 75, 80, 82, 91
resolution, 114, 120, 141
respiration, 73, 75
respiratory rate, 75
response, 38, 47, 48, 103
responsiveness, 41, 68
restrictions, 117, 133, 135, 138
retroperitoneal fibrosis, 129
RH, 109, 122
risk(s), 4, 15, 24, 25, 31, 32, 34, 36, 37, 39, 43, 57, 65, 68, 82, 88, 89, 93, 96, 102, 104, 105, 114, 121, 127, 129, 131, 133, 134, 135, 136, 137, 138
risk factors, 96
routines, 133, 135, 138
rubber, 24

S

safety, 31, 66, 67, 70, 79, 84, 86, 101, 137, 142
SAPS, 66
scope, 22, 23, 24, 25, 34, 40, 43, 80, 81, 82, 83
second generation, 139
security, 93
sediment, 12
semiconductor, 25
semirigid ureteroscope, 22, 24, 26, 40, 63, 64, 66, 70, 72, 128, 132
sensitivity, 113, 115, 117
sepsis, 128, 130, 135
sex, 35
shape, 8, 30, 43, 65
shock, vii, 3, 4, 14, 15, 16, 108, 117, 124, 125, 134, 139, 140, 141
shoot, 74
side effects, 38, 58, 115
signs, 36
silent hydronephrosis, 130
silica, 38
simulation, 142, 143
skin, 100, 101, 102, 103, 105
smooth muscle, 38
society, 131, 138
software, 142
solution, 37
speculation, 45
spinal anesthesia, 64, 73
spleen, 101
splint, 43
SS, 94, 96
stability, 69
staged URS, 135, 138
staghorn stone, 3, 8, 105
standard length, 30
state, 80
steel, 30, 41, 83
stenosis, 88, 101
stent, 12, 13, 29, 32, 43, 44, 45, 49, 55, 56, 57, 58, 60, 61, 63, 64, 65, 67, 68, 72, 80, 81, 84, 88, 89, 91, 92, 93, 95, 96, 97, 129, 130, 137
sterile, 37
stone basket, 19, 40, 41, 42, 43, 48, 67
stratification, 11
strictures, 44, 109, 131

structure, 40, 79
success rate, 12, 59, 133, 134, 135, 138, 139
surface area, 57, 90, 116, 118, 124
surgical intervention, 5, 113, 115, 116, 120, 129
surgical technique, vii
surveillance, 125
survival, 91
survival rate, 92
Switzerland, 101
symptoms, 5, 44, 45, 49, 55, 56, 61, 88, 89, 93, 95, 121

T

target, 73, 75, 82, 101, 105, 106
techniques, vii, 12, 22, 23, 37, 46, 63, 64, 75, 78, 104, 123, 127
technological advances, 13, 22, 25
technological progress, 81
technology(ies), 21, 29, 44, 45, 47, 122, 128, 133, 134, 142
tension, 30
therapeutic benefits, 128
therapeutic use, 21
therapy, 6, 13, 43, 54, 95
tissue, 37, 38, 131
titanium, 30, 41, 83
tones, 60, 134, 136, 138, 139
total internal reflection, 21
toxicity, 143
trainees, 75
training, 142
translocation, 130
transmission, 21, 22, 23, 24
trauma, 22, 30, 31, 38, 39, 40, 41, 68, 130, 131
trial, 5, 14, 15, 48, 62, 86, 94
tumor(s), 54,68
twist, 72

U

ultrasonography, 100, 101, 102, 103, 105, 107, 115, 123
ultrasound, 69, 80, 123, 131, 132
United States (USA), 56, 57, 88, 90, 100, 101, 122
urea, 91
ureter, 8, 12, 20, 22, 29, 31, 34, 37, 38, 41, 43, 44, 45, 46, 48, 54, 55, 56, 57, 58, 63, 64, 66, 67, 68, 69, 70, 71, 75, 79, 80, 81, 84, 89, 90, 93, 94, 101, 105, 106, 109, 128, 129, 141
ureteral stent, 43, 44, 45, 48, 49, 56, 57, 58, 59, 60, 61, 62, 63, 64, 65, 67, 68, 72, 80, 82, 84, 87, 88, 89, 91, 92, 93, 94, 95, 96, 97, 109, 129, 130, 137
ureteral stone, vii, 3, 4, 5, 8, 10, 11, 12, 40, 46, 48, 54, 59, 70, 71, 78, 79, 81, 82, 85, 88, 115, 117, 124, 130, 131, 134, 136, 137, 140
ureteral stricture, 35, 36, 44, 68, 70, 71, 72, 80, 84, 88, 91, 94, 120, 121, 131, 137, 142
ureteropelvic junction obstruction, 70
ureters, 29, 30, 32, 36, 44, 48, 57, 90, 93, 105
urethra, 46, 66, 67, 92
urinary tract, 13, 22, 24, 29, 34, 35, 38, 46, 47, 48, 53, 54, 59, 60, 62, 67, 69, 78, 80, 81, 116, 127, 130, 134, 136, 138, 139
urinary tract infection, 13, 53, 59, 62, 127, 130
urine, 12, 36, 37, 44, 84, 90, 127, 130
urologist, 36, 75
urothelium, 77
uterus, 20

V

valve, 20
variables, 57, 61, 89, 96
variations, 23
vasculitis, 34

vein, 57, 90
ventilation, 75
versatility, 78
vessels, 22, 35, 79
viscera, 79
vision, 40, 81
visual field, 36, 37
visualization, 22, 31, 34, 46, 58, 103, 106, 115, 116, 130, 135, 141
voiding, 45

W

water, 24, 38
well-being, 37

wires, 30, 31, 40, 41, 68, 75
withdrawal, 31, 40
worldwide, 78

X

xenon, 25

Y

yarn, 92
yttrium, 38, 124